Going Back to the Basics of Human Health

Avoiding the Fads, the Trends, and the Bold-Faced Lies

Completely Revised

Mary Frost

Copyright © 1997, 1999, 2004, 2007 by Mary Frost
Cover design by Joel Sharp

All rights reserved. No part of this book may be reproduced or transmitted in any form or by any means, including electronic or mechanical, without written permission of the author.

1st Edition
First Printing, 1997
Second Printing, 1997
Third Printing, 1998

2nd Edition
Fourth Printing, 1999
Fifth Printing, 2000
Sixth Printing, 2003

3rd Edition
Seventh Printing, 2004
Eight Printing, 2005

4th Edition
Ninth Printing, 2007

Published and distributed by
Expansive Health Awareness, Inc.
P.O. Box 178432
San Diego, CA 92177-8432
Phone: 619-276-2550   FAX: 858-274-9077
www.theperfectcrime.com   e-mail: mary@theperfectcrime.net

ISBN 978-0-9795038-0-1
Health and Fitness

Printed in the United States of America

To Dr. Royal Lee who was, and still is, a beacon of light for all of us who want to be healthy and stay healthy.

To my husband, Doug, who tirelessly supported me throughout the writing and multiple revisions of this book.

To Dr. Robert Curry whose support and leadership over the years has inspired me.

To Dr. Freddie Ulan who has been so supportive of this book, and me and whose workshops have transformed my nutritional practice.

To Lynn Irons and Peter Buckles for their brilliant consulting.

To the International Foundation for Nutrition and Health whose main goal is to educate people in the use of whole food nutrition. To John Brady III, Director, and all of the staff at the Foundation for their support.

To Dr. Michael Dobbins for conveying his scholarly study of Dr. Royal Lee's work in his nutritional seminars.

To Mo Rafael for her incredible book editing.

Author's Note

The following principles have guided my writing:

- *I don't claim to know everything.*
- *You and I are always learning.*
- *This book is in pursuit of the truth*
- *This book is a compilation of numerous medical and nutritional studies as well as many other resources that provide information relating to our health*
- *You and I are fellow travelers on the road to health and wellness*

Mary Frost has a B.A. in Journalism from the University of Texas and a Masters of Arts and Liberal Arts from St. John's College (The Great Books Program). She has been actively involved in health and nutrition for 25 years and brings her experience and studies to the forefront as a nutritional journalist.

This book is intended for educational purposes only and should not be used as a guide for diagnosis or treatment of any kind.

Contents

Introduction

Why Whole Food Supplements?

Most of us are used to reading literature proclaiming the benefits of vitamins, then deciding what is wrong with us and heading to the health food store to buy what we have decided we need. Often, we end up buying a myriad of vitamins that we take but we are still not any healthier.

What's happening here?

I, too, was once a health food store junkie. I would spend hours standing in the aisles, reading labels and talking with the clerks. At the time I was suffering from frequent sinus infections (7 in two years) that always resulted in laryngitis. I ended up taking vitamin A (25,000 IU), vitamin E (400IU), ascorbic acid with rose hips (3,000 mg.), Kyolic garlic, echinacea, goldenseal, and homeopathics but they did not help. I kept getting sick and, truthfully, was afraid that my immune system was getting so weak that I would end up dying from pneumonia (which I had already experienced three times in my late teens and early 20s).

I also did try seeing different health professionals, but with no result. Finally, I found an astute health professional who determined the underlying cause of my health problem and got me started on whole food supplements from a company called Standard Process. Using these whole food supplements, I got well and have stayed well. Today, if I start to get the sniffles, I immediately start taking some whole food supplements and I'm quickly over them. Before, I would take all the products I had purchased from the health food store, and I would still get sick.

Going Back to the Basics of Human Health

What I have come to realize over the years is that we cannot understand what any company offers us in the way of nutritional supplements unless we understand what has happened, step-by-step, to our food supply. And we cannot understand what a whole food supplement is offering us unless we understand what most vitamins today really are—synthetic. This means that the vitamin B you just picked up at your health food store or drugstore is probably derived from coal tar. It's easy for the manufacturer to claim it's "natural," because it once was—about 355 million years ago—but I like my vegetables a little fresher than that, and I know my body does too.

For decades Americans have gotten used to advertising that promotes the continually reoccurring concept of "new and improved." But, the truth is, we really don't know what that means. We don't step back and evaluate all the information that is being foisted upon us day after day because we assume it's true. One day we're told not to eat butter, but to eat margarine instead. Twenty years (and how many heart attacks) later we are finally told that margarine contains trans fats and is dangerous for us. We are told not to eat eggs or beef because they can cause cholesterol problems. Years later we are told that they are beneficial.

We are presented with "new medical facts" all the time, but what we are really getting is what Ralph Nader calls "pseudo-science." We are getting genetically modified foods, faulty infomercial tips, incorrect information about what we should be eating, and tricky nutritional labels we often have no way of deciphering.

Advertisements persuade us to change our eating habits and go in yet another dietary direction, but we need to stop listening to "those television advertising managers practicing medicine without a brain," whom Dr. Bernard Jensen and Mark Anderson refer to in their book, *Empty Harvest.* We need to stop running from one direction to another.

What I have attempted to do in *Going Back to the Basics of Human Health* is to pull back the subterfuge and take a look at the inner workings of this gigantic mess. Among other things, this book will explain why we need to tune out the antacid and low-fat diet commercials and why we must watch out for synthetic vitamins, either by themselves or hidden in any supplement. It is a guide to help us learn how to evaluate all of this confusing information and stay healthy.

Standard Process (the manufacturer of the whole food supplements I use) has always made its products available only through health professionals. If you are used to reading labels, their labels don't look anything like those on synthetic vitamin bottles. The sources are completely different, so the dosages are lower. But the people who have taken these whole food supplements for a period of time are repeatedly amazed at the improvement in their health and want to know more about how they work.

In the years I have been using whole food supplements I have seen amazing results with a variety of problems that people have presented to me. The therapeutic use of these whole food supplements really helps build people's immune systems and make them stronger and healthier.

But back in the days when I started taking whole food supplements, I was eating a low-fat diet and was tired and fatigued most of the time. I was introduced to Jay Robb's *Fat Burning Diet* and started eating a lot more protein. Within a short time I felt my life force coming back. It was then I realized the importance of blood sugar and optimal health. I read every book I could get my hands on that emphasized the importance of a high-protein diet, and I share some of this critical information in this book. For this revised edition I now offer the reader a glimpse into the completely unscientific history of how the low-fat diet rage got started.

I hope you will enjoy reading this book, and I trust it will open your eyes to the real health issues in America today. The process of gathering this information opened my eyes and changed my life forever. Here's to your health!

Going Back to the Basics of Human Health

Avoiding the Fads, the Trends, and the Bold-Faced Lies

"The U.S. spends more than twice as much per person on health care as 21 other industrialized countries. But our health ranks dead last (as measured by the World Health Organization's *Healthy Life Expectancy*: how many years of healthy life we can expect to live). It turns out that taking the most expensive drugs and having the most expensive procedures can be helpful or lifesaving sometimes, but for most people most of the time living a healthy lifestyle does far more to protect your health."

Dr. John Abramson, www.overdosedamerica.com

1/ Our Health Crisis Today

Every day we are bombarded with news stories or ads telling us just how sick we are. Celebrities like Patti La Belle have diabetes; Sally Field has osteoporosis; Brooke Shields took antidepressants. On top of that, we all know someone who has been diagnosed with a health problem. It could be cancer or heart disease, or any one of the new diseases being discovered on a regular basis.

Here are some often-quoted statistics:

- According to the American Heart Association, deaths from cardiovascular disease have gone from 28.9 % of all deaths in 2001 to 36.3 % of all deaths in 2004.
- The Centers for Disease Control (CDC) calls diabetes "disabling and deadly," and the number of people in the United States diagnosed with diabetes has more the doubled in the last 15 years.

- Roughly 25% of all adult Americans are obese. The CDC has called obesity an epidemic because it kills almost 500,000 people a year.
- According to the PBS program Critical Condition, which delved into the state of America's health care, more than 100 million Americans are chronically ill.
- More than 50 million Americans suffer from allergic diseases according to www.medicineworld.org
- Researchers at the University of Missouri say that approximately 50 million Americans have autoimmune disorders, involving a malfunction in the body's complex immune system.

Statistics like these can be intimidating. They can also make it seem like getting a disease is inevitable. Costs of orthodox medical treatment have skyrocketed, including drug costs, hospital costs, and insurance rates. Many experts say we are in a health crisis today and that medical costs could end up bankrupting our country.

In spite of all the money being pumped into orthodox medical treatments, the state of health care in the United States is getting worse. According to the American Public Health Association the average life expectancy is now dropping!

What To Do?

In an attempt to protect themselves and their families from frightening and serious health problems, many Americans are changing their diets and are taking herbs and supplements. It is estimated that one in three Americans seeks alternative treatment at a cost of $17 billion annually. Over-the-counter vitamin sales are at $6 billion per year. We pump vitamins and "eat right," yet good health continues to elude us. More Americans than ever before are fatigued, overweight, and depressed. Nearly every week Americans receive at least two or three mailers touting one new "medical breakthrough" after another. It was in response to this deluge of material that I have been urged to write this book—to enable people to wade through all this information and make informed decisions. There **are** solutions.

What Is Wrong With This Picture?

When people are trying so hard to do the right thing, why aren't the results long term? Why do they feel so great when they start taking vitamins and later feel fatigued again? Why are 95% of the people who lose weight unable to keep it off? Why are our national health statistics becoming alarming?

My studies have led me to conclude that there are three major culprits contributing to the disintegration of our health:

1. The harm that is done to our food before it even gets to us. The depletion and demineralization of America's topsoil; the contamination of produce by excessive use of pesticides, herbicides, and fungicides; the chemicalization of food through over-processing, enriching, and preserving; and the contamination of water from pesticide runoff and fluoridation.
2. Synthetic vitamins taken as supplements.
3. Low-fat, low-protein, high-carbohydrate diets.

Where Do We Start?

Foods are not what they once were. Despite its appearance, today's "fresh" produce is far less nutritious:

- To get the iron that was available in one cup of spinach in 1945, you would have to consume 65 cups today.
- An orange that contained 50 mg. of natural vitamin C complex in 1950 now contains 5 mg.

In most cases, that lovely green salad on your plate is practically dead nutritionally. "We are producing less nutritious food at the highest cost in history while United States farmers are going bankrupt."[1]

How can this be? It's simple to understand. There are three causes of America's topsoil depletion: deforestation, incorrect farming methods, and overuse of fungicides and pesticides.

Deforestation

Deforestation, while not in itself responsible for our nutritionally dead foods, marks the first major assault in the dismantling of our natural ecosystems. The cutting down of massive numbers of trees "laid bare" a disrespect for Mother Nature and a lack of interest in her inner workings.

When settlers began arriving in America in the 16th century, they found a land in pristine condition. After thousands of years of use by Native Americans, the water was still pure. The land was so fertile that if you dropped a seed it would grow. Trees and forests were everywhere. In fact, in the Iroquois Nation folklore they would speak of how a squirrel could hop from tree to tree from the Atlantic Ocean to the Mississippi River. When they gave directions "grandfather trees" were used as landmarks.

Today we are lucky to have any pure water, topsoil or forests at all. According to the U.S. Environmental Protection Agency in 1990, agricultural pollutants contaminate nearly half the wells and all of the surface streams in this country.

As for topsoil, a thin mantle of topsoil is the basic foundation of all civilization. Most scientists agree that it takes centuries, sometimes thousands of years for one inch of topsoil to form. However, the USDA has come up with a default position that soil forms at a rate of 1 inch per 30 years. Even with these contradictory views, according to the U.S. Global Change Research Information Office, "In the USA, soil has recently been eroded at **17 times** the rate at which it forms:

about 90 % of U.S. cropland is currently losing soil above the sustainable rate."[2]

The Europeans who settled in this country in the 1700s found 18 to 25 inches of rich topsoil! This is staggering. Topsoils in Iowa that were once a foot deep are now less than 6 inches deep. Dozens of studies analyzing the effect of erosion on land productivity found that the loss of one inch of topsoil reduces corn and wheat yields an average of 6%.

The causes of topsoil loss include ploughing too deeply, failing to rotate crops and grazing too many animals on the land. The hallmark of industrial agriculture—fence-to-fence plantings of only one crop with no hedges, trees or grasses around the edge of fields—is a big contributor. The soil then either blows away or is washed away because there is no vegetation to protect it.

Wind erosion in the Great Plains brought about the Dust Bowl of the 1930s and today "Wind erosion is a serious problem in the United States and the world. It is responsible for about half of the more than two billion tons of soil lost from U.S. cropland annually." [3] Water erosion is now the biggest cause of topsoil loss in the Great Plains and prior to 1985 cost Iowa almost 20 tons of topsoil for every three acres. Fence-to-fence plantings of one crop without the protection of diverse plantings, grasses, and trees have left the soil vulnerable to rain.

To date, over 260 million acres of trees in America have been cut to make way for raising livestock. Trees shade the soil, hold it in place, and act as pumps to draw water up near the surface of the ground thus keeping water tables high. Famine in countries like Ethiopia is due to deforestation. In the 1950s forests covered 16% of Ethiopia's total land area. Today only 4.2% remain.

U.S. Department of Forestry experts maintain that a country needs at least 10% of the land covered by forests. Today America's last forest reserves, our national parks, are threatened by adjacent mining activities, clear-cutting, and oil and gas exploration.

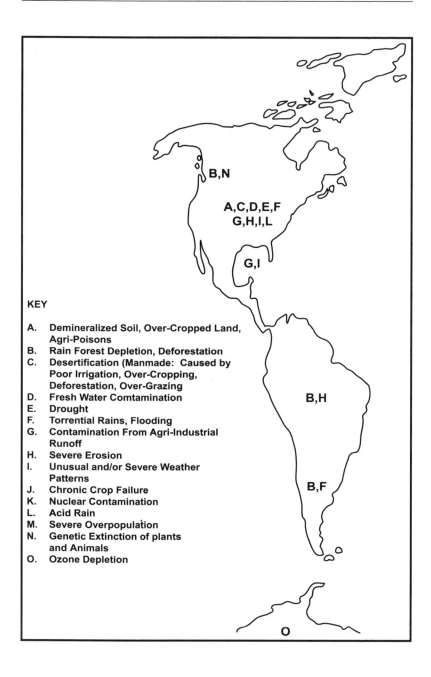

B,N

**A,C,D,E,F
G,H,I,L**

G,I

KEY

A.   Demineralized Soil, Over-Cropped Land,
     Agri-Poisons
B.   Rain Forest Depletion, Deforestation
C.   Desertification (Manmade: Caused by
     Poor Irrigation, Over-Cropping,
     Deforestation, Over-Grazing
D.   Fresh Water Comtamination
E.   Drought
F.   Torrential Rains, Flooding
G.   Contamination From Agri-Industrial
     Runoff
H.   Severe Erosion
I.   Unusual and/or Severe Weather
     Patterns
J.   Chronic Crop Failure
K.   Nuclear Contamination
L.   Acid Rain
M.   Severe Overpopulation
N.   Genetic Extinction of plants
     and Animals
O.   Ozone Depletion

B,H

B,F

O

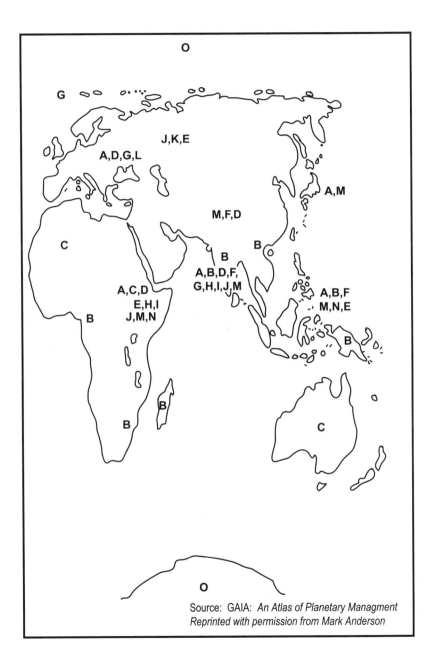

Source: GAIA: *An Atlas of Planetary Managment*
Reprinted with permission from Mark Anderson

Incorrect Farming Methods

The massive use of chemical fertilizers, which are manufactured and shipped around the world by the millions of tons per year, has come to be an accepted method of forcing plants to grow. This method was conceived in a paper published in 1855 by the renowned German chemist, Baron Justus von Liebig, who determined that the only minerals plants really needed were nitrogen, phosphorus and potassium.

The German chemical industry flourished on this premise by aggressively marketing it to farmers. The imbalance in trace minerals, fungus and microbial life that this "artificial manure" created was later regretted by von Liebig. At the end of his life he wrote, "Nature herself points out to man the proper course of proceeding for keeping up the productiveness of the land."[4]

Twenty years after von Liebig's death, the famed German naturalist, Julius Hensel, ridiculed this nitrogen-phosphorus-potassium theory in his book, *Bread From Stones*, and encouraged farmers to spread a finely crushed, mineral rich rock dust on their land. "Those who did were amazed at the quality, strength, and drought resistancy of their crops."[5]

The thriving chemical industrialists were so vicious and vigorous in their attempts to discredit Hensel that his book could not be found anywhere for many years. Their high-handed techniques illustrate how an idea that goes against the economic interests of the time can be squelched with such ferocity that people can actually conclude that it was false.

In 1940 Sir Albert Howard published his landmark book, *An Agricultural Testament*. In it he promoted Hensel's rock dust theories and gave a sober warning about the use of chemical fertilizers: "The principle followed, based on the von Liebig tradition, is that any deficiencies in the soil can be made up by the addition of suitable chemicals (man-made). This is based on a complete misconception of plant nutrition. It is superficial and fundamentally unsound. It takes no account of the life of the soil, including mycorrhizal association—the living fungus bridge which connects the soil and sap. Artificial manures lead inevitably to artificial nutrition, artificial food, artificial animals and finally, to artificial men and women." [6] You can't patent rock dust or manure and make immense profits from them.

Advocates of chemical fertilizers always argue that a plant really doesn't recognize the difference between a synthetic chemical and an organic source anyway. True. It doesn't. So what's the problem? The soil recognizes the difference.

A healthy vital population of organisms needs to be present in the soil in order to make all nutrients available to the plant. Hence the old adage, "Feed the soil, not the plant." Because synthetic chemical fertilizers are highly concentrated it is very easy to make a mistake with them. They need to be applied very **carefully** and with sound judgment and with organic products to balance them out. But recurring problems with our foods and our environment tell us that this just isn't done.

For one thing, soils really need to be analyzed prior to application. Applying more phosphorus to soils if they already have an adequate supply can cause runoff of the excess into nearby rivers and lakes. Phosphorus runoff is poisoning the Florida Everglades. In 2006 the Great Lakes in Michigan were covered with green slime, the explosion of toxic algae due to excess phosphorus.

Over-application of chemical fertilizers, which by definition are salt-based, can also kill microbes in the soil by a buildup of salt content. This creates a circular dilemma, since the only way synthetic nitrogen is made available to the plants is by the microbes . . . that are now dead. As this cycle continues, the soil becomes more and more unproductive and the nitrogen leaches out causing excessive nitrate concentrations in underground water tables.

Salts are an issue. In 1989, the Nutrient Testing Laboratory (NTL) ran mineral analysis tests on commercial produce from different regions in the United States. When the NTL compared them to charts from 1949, they found that sodium content had increased significantly over the last 40 years.

People are often fooled by the abundant, lush growth that synthetic fertilizers can cause in plants. But growing too fast can make the plants weak and the least wind or the most gentle spring rain can cause them to fall over. The lush growth can cause the plant to suck up more water, wasting that valuable resource, and it also makes them more attractive to insect pests.

Fungicides and Pesticides Are Not Working

Because farming has become a high-tech industry, combining technology and economics to exploit the land for profit, the result is that, "Modern agriculture reduces the role of soil to a substance of convenient texture that holds plants in the vertical position while chemicals are forced up their shaft."[7]

The modern corporate farmer is out of touch with the earth. He no longer gets down on his hands and knees and examines the soil. Instead, he looks at it from the heights of the air-conditioned cab on his $100,000 John Deere tractor. If he spots a fungus growing on a plant, he knows just what to do.

"He gets into his pickup truck, heads down to the agriculture chemical supply station and returns loaded with barrels of chemicals with skull and crossbones on their labels. Now he is ready to treat the plant. In the back of his pickup truck are barrels with labels that say things like: 'Use extreme caution—do not inhale—use in well-ventilated areas—do not allow any contact with skin and hair—do not dispose of near water—keep away from livestock and feed—may cause blindness or death if taken internally—read all instructions carefully—federal law requires application in accordance with label data.'"[8]

Totally oblivious to all of these warnings, the farmer applies these poisonous chemicals to our growing food! But we are just as oblivious, with absolutely no idea of how many different poisons are applied to our food. For years we have been told that **without** these chemicals we would have famine, so out of fear we have accepted them. But the truth is that industrial agriculture could be heading us toward famine.

Land that once was fertile in the Mississippi Delta is so devoid of worms and microbial life (signs of a healthy soil) that the remains of harvested crops cannot be turned under anymore. Years and years of soil sterilization have made the soil incapable of even rotting or composting.

According to Professor David Pimental, Department of Entomology at Cornell University, pesticide production from 1945 to 1990 increased an insane 3,300%. In the same time period crop loss due to insect damage increased 20%. This is because insects are mutating so as to be able to live on these poisons. The truth is pesticides are failing miserably and they are poisoning our food chain. And . . . we are not able to mutate as fast as insects do.

One deadly form of pesticide, *Zyclan B*, was used by the Nazis to gas millions of their victims in concentration camps from 1939 to 1945. Another, *Methyl Isocyanate*, killed over 3,500 people in Bhopal, India and maimed 200,000 more.

Now the oceans are being ruined by the runoff of chemical fertilizers, pesticides, and animal waste. All areas of the earth's oceans have always contained a wide variety of life. However, there are currently areas known as "dead zones," where the oxygen levels are so low that **no** marine life can live in them. According to OCEANA, one such "dead zone" forms in the Gulf of Mexico each spring and summer from the toxic runoff of the Mississippi River and covers almost 8,000 square miles, or an area the size of the state of Massachusetts.

Pesticides are difficult to eliminate. Pesticide residues can be found in plants grown in soil previously sprayed years before. Note the rigorous standards organic farmers must meet in California: No chemical fertilizers, pesticides or fungicides can be used on the land for three years, and the land is built-up organically. At the end of those three years, the produce is tested for pesticide residue. If there is any residue, the farmer must wait another year and have his product tested again before he can label it "Certified Organic."

You would think that, once it was understood that increasing the amounts of pesticides not only doesn't stop crop damage but actually increases it, the U.S. Government would have stepped in to protect us and stop all this nonsense. Not so. Instead, chemical companies have been allowed to go crazy, genetically manipulating crops in order to sell even **more** pesticides. *Mother Jones* Magazine published a chilling article in its Jan/Feb 1997 Issue, titled "The Future of Food," which told of potato and corn seeds that are genetically altered to contain a built-in pesticide and soybean seeds that are genetically manipulated to survive direct applications of the toxic herbicide Roundup™.

An article in the *New Yorker* magazine (April 10, 2000) traced the spread of genetically modified (GM) crops this way: "A decade ago, no transgenic crops were commercially available anywhere on earth; in 1995 four million acres had been planted; by 1999, that number had grown to one hundred million. In the United States, half of the enormous soybean crop and more than a third of the corn crop are products of biotechnology." [9]

Because GM crops like soybeans initially produce high yields they flood the marketplace and prices drop. The U.S. Government then comes to the rescue by paying out billions of dollars in subsidies to soybean farmers. This subsidy "help" actually hides the huge biotech research costs that should have made the GM soybeans more expensive. How does this play out in our lives? Now that soybeans are cheap, the processed food industry decides to promote soy as the new "miracle food" and puts GM soy into more than 30,000 food items. Basically, GM foods are then forced on the consumer by making it difficult for people to avoid eating them. Because there is such a huge disconnect between consumers and our agricultural system most of us don't even know this has happened.

Soil Is A Living Substance

Soil is the basis of all life. The plants that grow in soil are at the lowest end of the food chain and they in turn become food for animals at the next level of the food chain. These animals are then the food supply for humans at the highest end of the chain.

William Albrecht, PhD, Professor of Soils at the University of Missouri found that he could cure the disease undulant fever in livestock and humans simply by adding trace minerals to the soil in which their food was grown (Henry Ford's only son Edsel died from undulant fever). "When we see a symptom in the plant, it will always correlate to a poison or deficiency in the soil: when we see a disease in the human, it will relate to a poison or deficiency in the food."[10]

Dr. Albrecht's studies in the 1950s proved beyond a doubt that plants can appear healthy but have low quantities of nutrients. He also proved that the health of a plant is its own protection against insects. When a plant is healthy it has no need for pesticides whatsoever.

The early nutritionists and Dr. Albrecht were adamant that mineral-deficient soil is one of the original sources of disease in the world today. "Simply stated, food crops grown on depleted soil produce malnourished bodies, and disease preys on malnourished bodies."[11]

How Does A Plant Protect Itself?

What high-tech farmers are lacking is true understanding of a plant's immune system. In the plant's root system there are little offshoot rootlets that have hair-like fungi called *mycorrhizae* growing on them.

Good soil is composed of 45% minerals and is full of microbial life, which contains millions of bacteria. The bacteria's primary job is to decompose anything that falls on the land and to break down mineral deposits into plant food. The plant isn't devoured by the bacteria because the *mycorrhizae* secrete antibiotics to protect the plant. (Keep in mind that penicillin comes from a fungus.)

"Nature gave fungi and bacteria an interesting relationship.

They are natural antagonists. They keep each other in check through their competition. . . .The plant, thus protected, is free to absorb the minerals that soil microbial life has released without fear of infection from soil-borne bacteria." [12]

If we see a fungus growing on a plant, it is a self-produced fungus because there was something inferior about the quality of the plant. Nature grows a fungus on an inferior plant, which then dies, decomposes, and begins again—until it gets it right.

The Importance of Trace Minerals

"Human bodies require nutrition found in the form of plants, meat, milk and eggs." [13]   Since animals get their food directly or indirectly from plants and plants get their food from the soil, there is a direct link from the soil to human health.

Plants do not manufacture trace minerals, they **absorb** them. Much is said now in the news of the importance of different trace minerals, such as selenium, boron, and chromium. Just the absence of one trace mineral can cause health problems:

- Without the trace mineral cobalt, the human body cannot manufacture vitamin B_{12}.
- Without potassium, the heart muscle can be harmed and the result can be a "racing heart" or tachycardia.
- Without zinc, selenium, sulfur and iron, the liver would be sluggish and weak in its abilities to repair damaged tissue, fight infection and detoxify the blood and the bowel.

Also dependent on trace minerals are enzymes. All metabolic processes at the cellular level depend on enzymes. Sometimes called the "spark plugs of life," enzymes sustain, assimilate and transform all life processes through their catalytic action. No species can ingest food without the presence of enzymes. Often enzymes vital to our immune systems need the rarest trace minerals in order to function. There are 92 known trace elements.

As research continues, it is reasonable to assume that the role of every mineral will be discovered.

Let's Get Real

As we drive in our air-conditioned cars to our air-conditioned offices and sit down in front of our computers—only to go home at night and then sit in front of the TV—we are prey to an assault of information unparalleled in history. Yet, so much of what we hear does not take total, factual information into account.

The advocates of whole foods and organic farming are so out-talked by the advocates of big business that we can hardly hear the truth through all of their blaring. But our bodies know what is happening. The innate intelligence in our bodies is telling us through heart disease, cancer, AIDS, diabetes, and obesity that something is amiss. And our souls are telling us that profits aren't everything.

"Although the popular ecology movement grabs an occasional headline, what our political leaders, scientists and doctors are unwilling to come to grips with is that we are on the threshold of vast human annihilation. The effect to revitalize the human immune system must begin with a massive effort to return vitality and fertility to our soils." [14]

Consider what historian V.G. Simkovich had to say about the ruins of ancient civilizations: "Look at the unpopulated valleys, at the dead and buried cities, and you can decipher there the promise and the prophecy of us. . . . Depleted of humus by constant cropping, land could no longer reward labor and support life, so the people abandoned it. Deserted, it became a desert; the light soil was washed by the rain and blown around by the shifting winds." [15]

There is a possibility to reverse this trend. John D. Hamaker, in his monumental work, *The Survival of Civilization*, gives us some guidelines. Hamaker believes that "an all-out global effort to remineralize the Earth's soils (with rock dust) and the planting of billions of trees, coupled with the elimination of fossil fuel burning, and the development of alternative sources of power (for example, hydrogen, solar and wind) can restore the carbon balance between the land the atmosphere." [16]

The Chemicalization of Foods

Hmm. . . . Let's see now. Hundreds of millions of acres of trees have been chopped down, millions of acres of natural vegetation have been overgrazed, endless gallons of chemical fertilizers have been poured recklessly on the soil and untold amounts of fungicides and pesticides have been sprayed on plants. So, what's left in our food supply to be attacked? Why, natural foods, of course! Let's destroy all the enzymes left in them so they can sit on the shelf indefinitely.

As we navigate through the aisles at a grocery store, many of us have never noticed that it really is like a journey through a chemical laboratory. Some of us read labels, looking for one or two items on a list of ingredients that we are told contain additives, preservatives and synthetic vitamins. We take all this for granted and assume that what we are buying is still really food. The shocking truth of how all these substances came to be in our foods is not fully understood but should be.

Within a generation following World War I, the "foods of commerce" took over the marketplace. "The food supply became bleached, refined, chemically preserved, pasteurized, sterilized, homogenized, hydrogenated, artificially colored, defibered, highly sugared, highly salted, synthetically fortified (enriched), canned, and generally exposed to hundreds of new man-made chemicals." [17]

How did this happen? The first Food and Drug Law of 1906 was sabotaged from its very inception by commercial interests who had great influence within the U.S. Department of Agriculture (USDA). By 1912 they succeeded in forcing Dr. Harvey W. Wiley from his office as the head of the USDA's

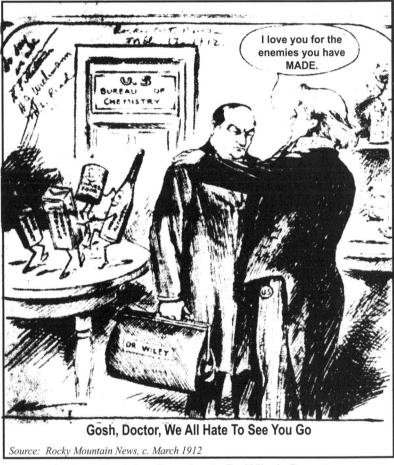

Gosh, Doctor, We All Hate To See You Go

Source: Rocky Mountain News, c. March 1912

Cartoon Depicting Reaction to Dr. Wiley's Departure
from the Bureau of Chemistry

Above: As Dr. Wiley prepares to leave, you can see on the table behind him caricatures of impure foods, patent medicines, and ersatz (synthetic) substances, all holding hands and dancing for joy. In the foreground, Uncle Sam bids farewell and laments the end of Dr. Wiley's career at the Bureau of Chemistry.

Photo and caption by permission of Mark Anderson

Bureau of Chemistry. They accomplished this by making it impossible for Dr. Wiley to do his job. It was the Bureau of Chemistry that had been given full authority by the law to decide what a violation of the law was and Dr. Wiley was considered too much of a purist.

He ordered the seizure of a shipment of bleached flour because the bleaching process left nitrate residue in the flour. The case of the *U.S. vs. Lexington Mill and Elevator Company* went all the way to the Supreme Court, which ruled **in favor** of the government and ordered the flour to be destroyed. But the head of the USDA, Secretary James Wilson, ignored this decision. Dr. Wiley commented that, "so far as bleaching flour is concerned by any process whatever, the Food and Drugs Act does not exist. The very law that the Supreme Court has said was en-acted to chiefly protect the public health has been turned into a measure to threaten public health and defraud the purchaser." [18]

Dr. Wiley also filed suit against Coca Cola™ to keep this artificial product off the market and prohibit its interstate transport. Explaining the rationale behind this lawsuit he said, "No food in our country would have any trace of benzoic acid, sulfurous acid or sulfites or any alum or saccharin, save for medical purposes. No soft drink would contain caffeine or theobromine. No bleached flour would enter interstate commerce. Our foods and drugs would be wholly without any form of adulteration and misbranding. The health of our people would be vastly improved and the life greatly extended. The manufacturers of our food supply, and especially the millers, would devote their energies to improving the public health and promoting happiness in every home by the production of whole ground, unbolted cereals and meals." [19]   (*Unbolted* means that the flour is not sifted, therefore the wheat germ is not lost.)

As you can see from the cartoon on the previous page, Dr. Wiley's departure was seen as an open frolic for the synthetic food enhancers. It marked the end of a unique period in our history, with a man of superlative training and great moral character at the head of decision-making regarding our foods.

A Dark Period for the FDA Begins

After Dr. Wiley's departure, the Bureau of Chemistry was gradually dismantled. By 1931 it had evolved into the Food and Drug Administration (FDA). From 1939 to 1949 teams of "experts" headed by the FDA's Dr. Elmer M. Nelson were in and out of federal court getting court orders to block health food manufacturers from telling the public what the difference was between the quality of their products and those of their synthetic, over-processed, counterparts. In other words, a manufacturer of whole-wheat flour was blocked from publicizing that white flour had lost 30 different nutrients.

Amazingly, the FDA's case rested on testimonies like the following one made by Dr. Nelson: *"It is wholly unscientific to state that a well-fed body is more able to resist disease than a less well-fed body.* My overall opinion is that there hasn't been enough experimentation to prove dietary deficiencies make one more susceptible to disease."* [20]

Unbelievable? Incredible? Is this true science? How many people today know that dietary deficiencies lead to degenerative diseases, infectious diseases, and functional diseases? The American public has been used as the official testing "lab" for this kind of fallacious thinking. It was these courtroom scenes, far away from the public eye, that set the stage for ruined, devitalized food to "legitimately" dominate the marketplace.

It is important to note that the landmark works in nutrition by Dr. Weston Price, Dr. Francis Pottenger, Dr. Roger Williams, Dr. Agnes Fay Morgan, Dr. Royal Lee, and others were totally ignored and treated with disdain. Also ignored was this statement from *Food & Life: The United States Department of Agriculture Yearbook for 1939*: "The chief fault of many American diets is that they provide too little of the essential minerals and vitamins. This fault is due in large measure to the fact that refined foods are consumed in such amounts that the intake of mineral and vitamin-rich foods is lower than it should be." (This publication is available at www.ifnh.org.)

The truth was helpless in the face of an FDA that had unlimited taxpayer dollars at its disposal to promote the commercial interests of the time. We need to understand that the United States Government has been controlled by special interests like the commercial food industry for nearly 80 years, and people today are just beginning to realize the dangers of this.

The Persecution of Dr. Lee

In the front lines of those who realized what was happening to our foods stood Dr. Royal Lee, a genius who applied his talents to finding solutions for all sorts of challenges. A prolific inventor, he came to hold 70 patents, mainly for electric motors and speed governors. But nutrition was his true passion.

He began showing an interest in nutrition at age 12. Later, while writing his senior paper in dental school he found research "which showed that tooth decay was most prevalent in youngsters with a high incidence of childhood diseases and non-existent in children who had been free of sickness. . . . After writing this paper, he was convinced that one of the most urgent problems facing humanity was to determine how to combat deficiency diseases. This became his lifelong passion and crusade." [21]

As his engineering company became successful Dr. Lee was able to take time to pursue his study of food chemistry. He began making concentrates of all major vitamin complexes, which he tested on himself and his family with phenomenal results. Dr. Lee felt he had a duty to help others and out of this was born a whole food supplement company (today known as Standard Process). Very quickly, his products met with greater and greater demand. In order to produce large batches for mass distribution that would still retain all of the vital nutrients, he designed high-vacuum, low-temperature dryers and special grinding mills.

When Dr. Lee tried to advertise and promote his supplements, the FDA took him to court over and over again. For example, in 1937 when Dr. Lee tried to advertise Zypan™ (the hydrochloric

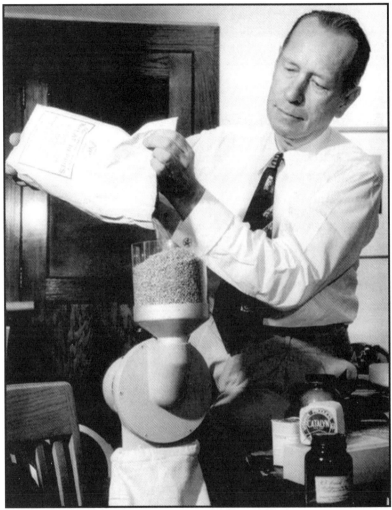

Dr. Royal Lee (1895 - 1967)

Perhaps the world's greatest nutritionist, Dr. Lee was also a prolific electronic inventor. Here he is working on his famous Lee Flour Mill. He designed it so the average household could have wholesome, fresh, low-heat, stone-ground flour with vitamin-rich germ and fiber-full bran intact. The Lee Foundation for Nutritional Research was a lighthouse as food adulteration and commercialism swept the twentieth century.

Photo and caption by permission of Mark Anderson

acid tablet he had designed to help with digestion), he faced competition from—of all things—cigarettes! The FDA ultimately prevented Dr. Lee from promoting Zypan, at the same time that it allowed Camel cigarettes to advertise in *Life* magazine that smoking cigarettes improved digestion.

Empty Harvest reproduces an astonishing 1937 ad. It shows a Thanksgiving meal divided into five courses, with short blurbs on how smoking between each course will "help your digestion to run smoothly."[22]   A food editor, Miss Dorothy Malone, is pictured in one corner of the ad saying, "It's smart to have Camels on the table.   My own personal experience is that smoking Camels with my meals and afterwards builds up a sense of digestive well-being. . . . Enjoy Camels all you wish—all through the day."[23]

How many people were powerfully persuaded to smoke cigarettes because of advertising? How many people think, "If it's advertised, it's true?" How many people suffered from lung cancer and heartburn that followed this kind of advice?

Another ad pictured in *Empty Harvest* gives out similar questionable advice about sugar. This 1955 ad claims "Science shows how sugar can help keep your appetite—and weight— under control."[24]   This ad actually promoted elevating blood sugar to cut down on the sensation of hunger. Is it any wonder that diabetes has been on the rise ever since?

Because we are constantly told that science has made incredible advances in health and nutrition, we believe it to be true. But when we come to understand what has actually been done to our foods we get a much different picture. And when we truly realize how much misinformation about health and nutrition we have been fed over the years, we can't help but wake up.

Unfortunately,   " . . . in many instances—and health and nutrition is one—the past is full of deception and factual manipulation resulting in the inheritance of a tarnished view of scientific progress."[25]

The foods that most people buy today are actually **worse** than the ones that Dr. Lee and other pioneers, such as Drs. Weston

Price, Melvin Page, and Francis Pottenger tried to expose as the cause of rampant malnutrition in our nation. These pioneers' studies repeatedly proved that refined carbohydrates and sugars cause tooth decay, diabetes, arthritis and other degenerative diseases. They also blamed the epidemic of coronary heart attacks that began sweeping the nation in the early 1920s on the lack of vitamins and minerals in over-refined foods.

Because Dr. Lee tried to promote the therapeutic use of whole unadulterated foods in a supplement form he found himself branded as a racketeer and a quack by the FDA. Despite the findings of the USDA's own *Food & Life* publication and several national health surveys that proved malnutrition was rampant, the FDA claimed that supplements were "not needed because the ordinary diet supplies amounts greatly in excess of those needed for good nutrition." [26] Armed with the power to muzzle and gag whole food advocates, the FDA allowed the marketplace to become filled with unhealthy over-processed grains and cereals.

As we navigate through the aisles of the grocery store most of us have no concept of the battles fought—and lost—by the early pioneers in nutrition who wanted to keep over-processed, dead and devitalized foods from the marketplace by educating people not to eat them. We have no idea it was continual FDA enforcement in one form or another that made it possible for all the chemical-laced foods to be on the shelf today.

In the mid-1940s artificial vitamins came into vogue and were added to these grains and cereals, all for huge profits. "The *Nutrition Action* (Vol.16, No.1) reports that the only difference between General Mills' Wheaties and Total cereals is that 1.4 cents' worth of synthetic vitamins are sprayed on Total. Total is then sold for 65 cents more than Wheaties. This practice alone has generated $425 million in additional profits since 1972 for General Mills." [27]

Sadly, these huge profits mean that hundreds of millions of people have ingested untold pounds of chemicalized and enriched foods to their own detriment. The healthy world that Dr. Wiley, Dr. Lee and others had envisioned was not allowed to be.

The Altering of Oils

Today, sickness is always in the news. Because of this, it's hard for us to realize that "One hundred years ago, heart attacks were practically unheard of in the United States. . . . Alzheimer's disease did not exist. One person in 100,000 had diabetes. . . . One hundred years ago, people ate fresh, whole foods, including plenty of meat, butter, and lard. But they did not ordinarily eat any refined, processed or chemicalized foods, did not eat any refined and altered oils or fats." [28]

Most people don't realize that oils contain nutrients—when they are unrefined. Dr. Royal Lee pointed out in his lectures in the 1950's that natural fats and oils contain Vitamins A, E, K and trace minerals and that we need them to maintain our normal weight, normal blood pressure, to prevent heart disease, and to maintain our sexual characteristics. He warned of the destruction to our health when fats and oils are tinkered with.

Fats or oils from seeds are extracted by first grinding and then expeller pressing the seeds. When manufacturers wanted to increase the amount of oil produced, they applied solvents to the ground seed mixture to extract more oil, increasing the amount by almost 80%. Benzene was the first solvent to be used, but hexane is the one predominantly used today. Hexane is a high-vapor pressure component of gasoline that is easily ignited. Not surprisingly, the EPA lists it as a carcinogen.

The edible oil industry claims that all traces of hexane either evaporate or are removed in a "stripping column." However, studies done in 1997 by S.V. Overton and J.J. Manura on six cooking oils extracted with hexane found higher levels than expected of pentane, hexane, octane and benzene. (Yum!)

But the processing nightmare doesn't stop there. Many oils are hydrogenated, which means they are subjected to high heat, a metal catalyst, and hydrogen gas. Then they are degummed. This process removes chlorophyll, vitamin E, lecithin, minerals and trace minerals. If the oil is to be used for cooking it is then bleached. If it is to be used for salad dressings, will be refrigerated and needs to stay in an oil form, it is then "winterized," rapidly chilled and filtered to remove any waxes that still remain.

The final step is deodorizing by steam distillation at temperatures over 450 degrees F. This removes any unwanted tastes incurred by the earlier processing methods and insures the all-important goal . . . a longer shelf life.

We are used to seeing the end product of all of these processes as the colorless oils in clear plastic bottles displayed on shelves of grocery stores and health food stores. When we open them they don't have any real odor or taste, and now we know why.

Be sure to pick the oils you use carefully. Buy oils in cans or dark brown glass bottles and only oils labeled "cold pressed." Fresh natural oils have their own delicate aroma and flavor. At home, open your bottle of oil and smell it. If you detect even a whiff of rancidity, throw it away.

Enter Trans Fats

Most vegetable oils that are made from seeds cannot be used for baking and deep fat frying unless they are changed **again** from a liquid oil into a solid fat. When you try to substitute a cup of oil for a cup of butter or lard in your cookie recipe you will end up with a flat greasy cookie. Frying foods in unrefined oil can cause them to look greasy, and the oil spoils quickly.

These nasty problems are fixed by a process called "partial hydrogenation," which changes oils into man-made plastic fats that do not melt at room temperature (or at body temperature either). But who cares, when the baker can pack more fat into a product without a greasy feel or the restaurant that does a lot of deep fat frying can use the same oil over and over again because it is so resistant to heat damage?

This partial hydrogenation process has produced a whole new class of fatty acids called *trans fatty acids* that we are hearing so much about in the news today. The FDA has determined that the safe level of trans fats in the diet is ZERO. Instead of banning them from foods the FDA simply required the processed food industry to label all trans fat content, starting in 2006. (Buyer Beware: The FDA allows foods that list partially hydrogenated oil in the ingredients to say ZERO trans fats on the Nutrition Facts Label if they contain less than .5 grams per serving. This adds up, e.g., five cookies with .4 grams of trans fats = 2 grams.)

Not satisfied with this lack of enforcement, in December 2006 the New York City Board of Health voted to ban trans fats at restaurants in the city. "Restaurants will have to eliminate the artificial trans fats from all of their foods by July 2008." [29]

The FDA estimates the average American eats 4.7 pounds of trans fats each year. I think it's a lot more than that. Ten days of eating chicken nuggets (12-18 grams of tans fats), French fries (5-12 grams), and snack chips (6 grams) and you could easily be at 350 grams.

Some Very Real Dangers

Although the NYC Board of Health banned trans fats from foods because of their "artery-clogging" properties, there are other real problems we rarely hear mentioned. Dr. Mary Enig, one of today's foremost experts on the nutritional aspects of oils, reports that cellular damage caused by consuming trans fatty acids "correlates to low birth weight in human infants; increases blood insulin levels . . . increasing the risk for diabetes; affects immune response by lowering the efficiency of B cell response and increasing proliferation of T cells; precipitates childhood asthma." [30]

Think about it. The U.S. ranks 74th in the world in infant mortality due to low birth weight. Diabetes is becoming an epidemic. Immune disorders and childhood asthma are on the rise. Trans fats are about as dangerous to eat as any substance the food industry has ever created. We need to stop consuming trans fats for many reasons.

Water—A Vehicle for Drugs

In 1928 Dr. Royal Lee wrote a paper in which he "showed that tooth decay was greatest by far in children who had such poor nutrition that their resistance was lowered, not only to tooth decay, but also to all other diseases of childhood." [31]   Dr. Weston Price later irrefutably proved this link in his landmark work, *Nutrition and Physical Degeneration.* (See pp.46-49)

But in 1951 the U.S. Public Health Service (PHS) urged that fluoride be added to America's drinking water in order to prevent cavities. This set us off on a faulty track, looking away from malnutrition as the real cause. The book *Fluoridation: The Great Dilemma* (see Resources) traces the historical roots of this PHS decision to a problem that the Aluminum Company of America (ALCOA) and other manufacturers of aluminum cooking utensils began having in the early 1930's. It seems that a by-product of the smelting process, sodium fluoride, was nearly impossible to get rid of.

It couldn't be dumped in the ground because it caused serious contamination of grasses used for animal feed. When it was dumped in water, fish hatcheries were ruined and they sued aluminum manufacturers and won. An epidemic of lawsuits from cattlemen and farmers ensued. What to do? Pour money into research programs with the sole intent of creating a flood of favorable scientific reports to convince communities and the courts that small amounts of fluoride are not harmful to man.

In 1939 one scientist at the Mellon Institute, Gerald Cox, went one step further, claiming that humans **needed** fluoride for tooth formation and it should be added to water supplies as a means of reducing tooth decay. This set the tone for other aluminum-industry funded research, and the flood of pro-fluoride scientific papers ensued. Cox actively promoted the need (?) for fluoridated water to dental organizations like the American Dental Association and this "cutting edge" concept caught on.

The naturally occurring form of fluoride found in mineral-rich well water, calcium fluoride, was supposedly too costly to be used for this public "health" purpose. So guess what? Sodium fluoride became the source for the fluoride added to municipal drinking water. This started out as a 10-year experiment but, thanks to heavy lobbying, was left in place for decades.

Today 90% of the United States water fluoridation programs use fluosilicic acid, a classified hazardous waste derived from the "pollution scrubbing devices of the super phosphate fertilizer industry, 70 to 75% of which comes from the Cargill fertilizer corporation. The only other place this fluosilicic acid can be disposed of is a hazardous waste facility." [32]   At this facility it would cost $1.40 or more per gallon to be neutralized.

We need to become aware that we have allowed industries to promote the notion that fluoride prevents tooth decay in order to sell their toxic waste to our municipal water districts. Numbed by an overwhelming amount of industry-sponsored research, many of our politicians aren't bothered by the toxic sources that fluoride comes from. They won't even vote for bills that mandate fluosicic acid be tested for safety, in spite of the fact that the FDA has never approved fluosilicic acid as fluoride in the first place.

It is groups like the Fluoride Action Network and the Citizens for Safe Drinking Water that have warned us about fluosilicic acid and about its long-term side effects. For one, it depresses the thyroid, a problem affecting 20 million Americans. "Insufficient thyroid hormones cause all bodily functions to slow down . . .the symptoms of hypothyroidism are subtle and gradual and may be mistaken for depression." [33]   A study published in the *Journal of the American Medical Association* (JAMA) in 1990 concluded that drinking fluoridated water doubles the incidence of hip fractures in older men and women.

Sweden refused to fluoridate their water after consulting the Nobel Medical Institute. France consulted the Pasteur Institute and refused to fluoridate. Our water is being fluoridated against the best scientific advice in the world. It's up to you to protect your health against this toxic substance and drink purified water, checking to make sure the filtering process removes fluoride.

"I had a letter from an Austrian colleague who was
suffering from a severe hemorrhagic diathesis
(infection). He wanted to try ascorbic acid in
(for) his condition. Possessing at that time no sufficient
quantities of crystalline ascorbic acid, I sent him a preparation
of paprika that contained much ascorbic acid and the man was cured by
it. Later, with my friend, St. Rusznyak, we tried to produce the same
therapeutical effect in similar conditions with pure ascorbic acid, but
we obtained no response. It was evident that the action of
paprika was due to some other substance present in the plant."

Albert von Szent-Gyorgi
Hungarian-born U.S. biochemist; Nobel Prize winner
for discovering that vitamin C cured scurvy.

2/ Synthetic Vitamins vs. Food

The FDA has claimed for years that foods are not therapeutic. *Funk and Wagnall's* definition of *therapeutic* is "having healing qualities; curative." The early nutritional pioneers believed that whole foods were the **only** foundation for optimum health and, as such, were also the main foundation for a **return** to health. I agree with them. However, the dismissal of the therapeutic value of whole foods made it possible for the FDA and our lawmakers to support a commercial food industry whose sales today total more than $500 billion! It's no wonder that you and I are left with a health crisis that is out of control.

Attempting to help themselves, most people run to their local drugstore or health food store and grab some synthetic vitamins off the shelf. Or they may call on a friend or visit the web to get the latest cure from a multi-level marketing company, which usually claims that their product contains the latest isolated nutrient factor (synthetic, of course). But what all the marketers don't know is that in the long run they may be compounding their customers' health problems by encouraging them to take their companies' synthetic isolates as vitamins.

Most people take vitamins in the first place to replace what's missing in their foods. What they don't realize is that when they take synthetic vitamins they're really only getting more of what's already being dumped into their foods under the guise of enrichment. *Webster's Dictionary* defines "enrich" as "to improve the quality of; to make a valuable addition to." Take a look at a loaf of enriched bread...has it really been improved?

On the bread wrapper it will say "enriched flour (barley malt, ferrous sulfate (iron), "B" vitamins (niacin, thiamine mononitrate (B1), riboflavin (B2), folic acid)." *The Consumer's Dictionary of Food Additives* by Ruth Winter, M.S., states that ferrous sulfate is used as "a wood preservative, weed killer, and to treat anemia." Thiamine mononitrate is derived from coal tar. If you were to take a blowtorch to a B vitamin made from this substance it would turn into a glob of tar, much like the tar on your roof. And these are only two of the ingredients that are supposed to improve the quality of the dead white flour used to make bread.

How can anything made from coal tar be called a vitamin in the first place? How can taking a coal tar vitamin make up for what is removed from foods?

In truth, we should question **all** vitamins. As there is no specific definition for what constitutes a "natural" or an "organic" vitamin as far as the FDA is concerned, this kind of ambiguity leaves plenty of room for abuse by the unscrupulous.

To understand what we need to look for in vitamins, here are some explanations of terms based on both the sources and the processing used:

Natural – These are vitamins found in foods and not tampered with in any way that might change their molecules or their biochemical actions. Labels should indicate the exact food source the vitamin is obtained from.

Crystalline – These are vitamins taken originally from a food source and then treated with heat, caustic high-powered solvents (such as benzene or toluene), chemicals, and distillations to reduce them to a specific vitamin.

Synthetic – These are vitamins made in a laboratory that are chemically reconstructed versions of the crystalline vitamins from other known sources. Thiamine mononitrate made from coal tar is a synthetic vitamin. (Note: Chemists call everything that is derived from coal "organic" because it has carbon in its molecular structure.)

Why Natural Food Complexes Faded from View

When vitamins were discovered, they were discovered in foods. When foods were studied, a lot was learned. In fact, in the studies that showed that vitamins really do work, a food-source nutrient (such as wheat germ oil) was used. In studies showing that vitamins don't work, a synthetic (such as an alpha tocopherol vitamin E) was always used.

Since food nutrients tend to vary, they were difficult for an agency like the FDA to control. But synthetically isolated vitamins were easy to standardize and control. The measurements of milligrams or micrograms as "standards" of effectiveness were based on animal tests using isolated vitamin fractions, not foods.

Over the last 60 years conventional medicine has evolved into a tight-knit profession that largely ignores the downturn in the nutrient quality of our foods. The early nutritionists understood that these nutritionally dead foods were the main cause of disease through cellular malnutrition. But this line of thinking has been left out of conventional medicine. In her book, *The Real Truth About Vitamins and Antioxidants*, noted nutritional author Judith DeCava makes some important points:

- "Medical schools in this country are now standardized (if not homogenized) and no matter what medical school one attends, one gets essentially the same instruction." [34]

- In 1991 only 22 out of the entire 127 accredited U.S. medical schools required a single course in nutrition, which only 5% of the medical students actually took. Patients look to doctors for all kinds of advice and, though ill-prepared to offer advice in some areas, doctors seem to believe that they have a sort of supremacy to lend their expertise in areas of medicine for which they have received no training, "as in nutrition, leading them to discount ideas and even valid research." [35]

- From World War II onward, nutritional information has been based on research studies funded by the interests of the pharmaceutical companies which, (and this might surprise you) are **the** manufacturers of all crystalline and synthetic vitamins. "A few large pharmaceutical corporations such as Merck and Hoffman-LaRoche produce the crystalline-pure vitamin fractions used in virtually all nutritional supplements whether found in a drug store, health food store, or doctor's or nutritionist's office. Whole food complexes are just not as profitable." [36] Most vitamin fractions can be produced for pennies and sold for a few dollars and up. The profits are immense.

- Established medicine has based itself around the use of a large number of chemical substances (drugs), which appear to bring relief from specific symptoms. Synthetic vitamins, which have drug-like effects, are the only vitamins accepted by the majority of the medical profession . . . when vitamins are accepted at all.

Why Are Natural Complexes So Important?

Vitamins are "groups of chemically related compounds." In the case of vitamin C there is a single part identified as the organic nutrient, i.e., ascorbic acid as vitamin C. But there are enzymes, co-enzymes, antioxidants, trace elements, activators,

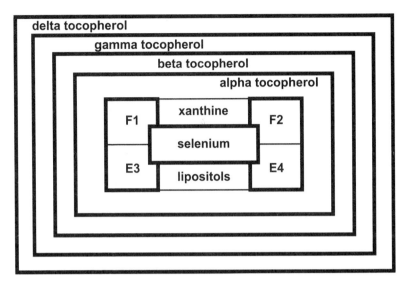

The Functional Architecture of the Vitamin E Complex

Reprinted with permission from Judith DeCava

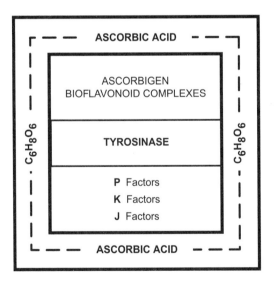

**The Functional Architecture
of Vitamin C Complex**

Reprinted with permission from Judith DeCava

33

and other **unknown** factors that enable the vitamin to go into bio-chemical operation. (See diagrams on the previous page.) In other words, ascorbic acid is only a part of the vitamin C complex. It is not, all by itself, vitamin C.

"With foods and food concentrates—containing whole nutritional complexes—the body can choose its needs for assimilation and excrete what it does not need; this is called 'selective absorption.' On the other hand, with fractionated or isolated and/or synthetic vitamins, there is no choice; the body must handle the chemical imbalances and toxic overdose." [37]

The natural vitamin complex of foods cannot be taken apart and reassembled and be expected to work the way it did before. It's not like a car or a watch; it's **alive**. In fact, when it's taken apart it won't work at all. Yet this is exactly what has been done to produce crystalline or synthetic vitamins.

The "scientific method" then takes these dead and inert vitamins and develops trials or experiments with them. DeCava sees this as unfortunate: "Synthetic, fractionated, crystalline-pure vitamins are not whole, natural compounds; they are not food which human systems can utilize as nutrients, with which human systems are familiar, and which will not disrupt normal biochemistry. How could any scientist say that the body does not know the difference between natural and synthetic vita-mins?" [38]

What has happened is that "true science is now judged on the basis of an experimental method which measures, classifies, and duplicates reactions and effects of single chemicals. This rules out testing natural vitamin complexes." [39] People do not understand that the rules and parameters for testing vitamins from the 1960s on pretty much eliminate the use of any natural food-based products. What have been used in "vitamin" tests are micro-parts of oils and coal tar that can be patented. You can't patent wheat germ oil or liver or yeast and make enormous profits.

Rats and the Recommended Daily Allowances (RDAs)

The "scientific" studies I just mentioned substitute dead synthetic or crystalline-pure vitamins for whole food complexes and then go on to ignore the human element by substituting rats, chicks and rabbits for humans. A zoo would never feed all their different animals the same food or the same proportions, yet the RDAs for humans are now based on Rat Bioassay.

"The bioassay method is based on the direct measurement of a vitamin's 'biological activity in preventing or curing certain specific pathological (disease) conditions in a predetermined experimental animal,' in most cases, the rat. This method 'expresses measurement, in terms of units.' So the amount found to alleviate disease in the rat or other laboratory animal is 'translated' into the amount and form needed for humans." [40]

But rats are scavengers. Humans are not. The physiological makeup of lower animals enables them to eat, digest and utilize foods and rubbish that we cannot. Take scurvy, for example. In *Taber's Cyclopedic Medical Dictionary* scurvy is defined as, "A deficiency disease [of vitamin C] characterized by hemorrhagic manifestations." Rats can convert ascorbic acid "into the required vitamin C complex. Such animals with scurvy, when fed ascorbic acid, may improve so that symptoms are relieved. Humans with scurvy, when fed ascorbic acid, do not improve very much, if at all." [41]   (This is what Szent-Gyorgi was discussing in the quote at the beginning of this chapter.)

In spite of the fact that rat studies don't really exemplify how humans utilize synthetic vitamins, the government has put into place standards that supposedly reflect "adequate" (synthetic) vitamin levels for individuals. The RDA for vitamin C is 60 milligrams per day. But according to DeCava, "many biochemists and nutrition scientists 'regard the government's recommended daily allowances (RDAs) of vitamins as inadequate for the prevention of chronic diseases." [42]   This is of major concern for all of us because chronic diseases are the ones that are slow to develop and can be long and drawn out.

For example, even though people don't get a classical vitamin C deficiency (scurvy) in this country, long before the telltale signs of scurvy manifest, a person could have all the signs of a marginal vitamin C deficiency: painful joints, easy bruising and gums that bleed with brushing of the teeth. These symptoms mean that the body's nutrient storages are gradually being drained and its health is being weakened, leaving it more susceptible to disease.

How many pain medication advertisements that you see weekly focus on people with painful joints? How many people do you know who complain of "bruising easily"? Vitamin C is just one vitamin that people are not getting adequate amounts of, and what they are getting in their synthetic vitamins and in their processed foods is obviously not doing the job.

Getting to the Heart of The Matter

Not only do synthetic or crystalline-pure vitamins not work, they're also not good for you. Why? It's very simple. They're not real and they can be harmful. For example, a person starts taking ascorbic acid. If he/she has sufficient reserves of the other components of the C complex (enzymes, co-enzymes, anti-oxidants, trace element activators and other unknown factors) to recombine and process their intake of pure ascorbic acid, that person will experience some improvement for a time. However, when these reserves are drained, the ascorbic acid will no longer benefit that person. The very symptoms that the person was trying to eliminate will return even while the person is still taking the ascorbic acid; and now the person will have a full-blown vitamin C deficiency.

The body treats all synthetic vitamins as foreign substances, reacting to them like toxins. These toxins are then processed and neutralized by the liver, which sends them to the kidneys for elimination. This is the real story behind the "expensive urine" of excess vitamin intake.

Many people feel an energy increase, even euphoria, when they start to take synthetic vitamins. But taking excessive amounts for an extended period of time will cause the effects to reverse. DeCava gives the example of taking synthetic B1, saying it "will initially allay fatigue but will eventually **cause** fatigue by the build-up of pyruvic acid. This leads to the vicious cycle of thinking more and more thiamine is needed, resulting in more and more fatigue along with other accumulated complaints." [43] Because people have widely differing amounts of stored reserves there are two facts that sincere nutritionists in whole food complex research keep trying to bring to our attention:

- Vitamins cannot be standardized, because there is no way to determine what different people's needs are and there is no way to calculate their reserves.
- Every individual's abilities to process, recombine and eliminate synthetic vitamins are difficult to gauge.

Whole Natural Vitamins vs. Synthetic Vitamins

Judith DeCava said it succinctly: "Regardless of the seemingly good initial response, using 'high potency' synthetic vitamins will, in time, bring a person into that 'intermediate zone' where the effects begin to reverse. This partially explains the confusion between natural and synthetic vitamins." [44] Ms. DeCava quotes numerous studies that compare natural vitamins to synthetic vitamins, and the natural ones always come out ahead. But how do we, as consumers, know what is natural and what is not?

The named source of the vitamin is our best clue. The chart on the next page allows you to compare the synthetic versus the food-based forms of some common vitamins. You might want to

VITAMIN	SYNTHETIC VITAMIN	FOOD-BASED VITAMINS
Vitamin A	Acetate Retinal Palmitate Beta Carotene	Fish oils Liver Carrot powder
Vitamin B_1	Thiamine HCl Thiamine Mononitrate	Nutritional yeast
Vitamin B_3	Niacin	Nutritional yeast, liver
Vitamin C	Ascorbic Acid Pycnogenols	Green leafy vegetables Buckwheat juice, citrus
Vitamin D	Irradiated Ergosterol	Cholecalciferol, fish oil
Vitamin E	d-Alpha Tocopherol dl-Alpha Tocopherol d-Alpha Succinate	Wheat germ oil Green leafy vegetables Peavine plant

make a copy of it to have on hand. When you're feeling brave, look in your cupboards and see how your foods stack up. Bear in mind that synthetic vitamins, which are **legally** considered to be equal in nutritional value to food-based vitamins, are far cheaper to make and therefore dominate our foods. We are also used to seeing listings in high milligram potencies. But a high number of milligrams is also an indication of a synthetic source.

The B vitamins are some of the most important vitamins our bodies need. Vitamins B and C are not stored in the body, so we must constantly replenish them. In nature, the B vitamins are always found together, one is never isolated from the rest. Consequently, the B vitamins should always be taken as a whole.

Dr. Royal Lee said in his *Vitamin News* that "a natural combination [of vitamin B Complex] is likely, according to clinical experience, to be from ten to fifty times more potent in humans, unit for unit, than is a chemically purified or synthetic complex, or a natural complex derived from only ONE source. No ONE source contains ALL the factors of the complete vitamin B complex, and for highest potency a number of therapeutically active sources must be tapped." [45]

Dr. Lee listed 22 factors and synergists in his B complex. By tapping into so many different food sources, he was able to include vitamin B_4, which he called the anti-paralysis factor. He said that a deficiency in vitamin E can result in muscle degeneration of the heart; a vitamin B_4 deficiency can cause a heart block due to the degeneration of the nerves in the heart muscle.

(People always consumed the entire vitamin B and E complexes when their cereal and bread grains were whole and contained the cereal germ. Today this is no longer true. Modern food processing changed all that by destroying these complexes and all the while telling us how healthy their foods were!)

Dr. Lee noted that the 22 different food factors and synergists in his vitamin B tablet combined into 50 to 100 isomers. For the chemist and the layperson, the molecular complexity of this is mind-boggling. All of this complex potency is lost when a vitamin is synthesized.

Standard Process lists on its Cataplex B bottle the following milligrams per three tablets. (*Cataplex* means whole food complex.):

Thiamine	0.95 mg
Niacin	20.44 mg
Vitamin B_6	0.95 mg

This product is a far cry from the majority of B complexes on the market, which list each synthesized B vitamin in a range from 50 to 100 mg. Cataplex B does not, however, list every B vitamin because the multitude of other B vitamin factors are present in small, potent, food-based amounts that the FDA has no approved labeling for. The FDA only recognizes milligrams based on synthetic vitamins (i.e., measurable chemicals).

What Is Potency?

DeCava explains the term *potency*: " . . . the strength, ability, or capacity to bring about a particular result . . . of vitamins 'measured' in milligrams or micrograms, based on test results on animals using isolated vitamin fractions." [46] "High potency" vitamins require a large amount of the fractured vitamin to achieve a specific reaction although, as previously mentioned, not necessarily a nutritionally beneficial reaction.

The reality is that a **minute** amount of a vitamin in its whole food form is more effective nutritionally than a large amount of a synthetic one! An excellent illustration of this is the story involving a medical doctor held captive in a prisoner of war camp during the Korean War (1950-1953). After a period of time on their severely inadequate diet, many of the doctor's fellow prisoners began showing signs of beriberi, a disease that results from a severe thiamine (B1) deficiency. He notified the Red Cross, and they sent him thiamine in a synthetic form, thiamine HCl (a coal tar-based vitamin). The doctor gave this to his patients, but their health continued to deteriorate.

Finally the doctor's North Korean guards whispered to him that beriberi could be cured with rice polish, the nutritive outer layers of the rice that are removed when it is refined. He thought the suggestion was absurd, but he had nothing to lose so he started giving his patients a teaspoon or more of rice polish every day. Within a short time, the beriberi epidemic ceased.

There is only about one level teaspoon of thiamine in an entire ton (2,000 ponds) of unrefined, whole rice. The amount of thiamine that the prisoners of war were getting in their rice polish was infinitesimal. What a tribute to unrefined rice and an excellent example of the potency of whole foods! How sad that vitamin-deficient white rice is the norm today and has ruined the natural immunity and health of millions of Asian peoples.

Synthetics Are Not As Effective

DeCava quotes study after study that proves synthetics just don't work. Here's the main reason why: With vitamin E we're used to seeing the tocopherol capsules. But when you take just the tocopherol, you've thrown out the real vitamin E because the tocopherols are nature's way of protecting and preserving Vitamin E; similar to the way the peel of a banana protects the contents. Vitamin E actually **"loses up to 99% of its potency when separated from its natural synergists."** [47]

Taking the synthetic version of vitamin E can actually be quite harmful. "In one test study, the vitamin E-deficient laboratory animals fed tocopherols died sooner than the control animals that received no vitamins at all." [48]

Taking synthetic B vitamins exclusively can be dangerous, too. "Silver foxes were fed a synthetic diet so that every component of the diet would be known. The animals were given all of the known B vitamins—in synthetic form—but they did not grow; their fur deteriorated, and finally they died. Another group of foxes on the same diet were given a change after a short time: added to their rations were yeast and liver, both sources of natural whole B complex. These animals grew normally and the quality of their fur improved with their health." [49]

Many people reach for ascorbic acid when they have a cold. Yet "modern-day studies, utilizing ascorbic acid (the crystalline-pure fraction) rather than vitamin C complex, find the synthetic fraction has virtually no effect on pneumonia, bronchitis, or other pulmonary problems even though sufferers show low serum levels of vitamin C . . . daily intake of ascorbic acid supplements reduces the total white blood cell count, compromising the immune response rather than assisting it." [50]

Confusion about ascorbic acid is created by reports of how it has helped to fight colds and infections in short-term use. *Empty Harvest* points out that, "the answer probably lies more in ascorbic acid's pH balance influence (acid/alkaline balance) than any other factor." [51]

Since most infectious bacteria thrive in an alkaline pH, high consumption of ascorbic acid when first catching cold creates an acid environment in which the bacteria can't thrive. In his book *Folk Medicine*, Dr. D.C. Jarvis stressed the importance of the acid/alkaline balance in the body's immune system and recommended that people take 2-3 tablespoons of apple cider vinegar daily to acidify their systems. Apple cider vinegar is a whole food that is 5% acetic acid, which is normally found in the body. Taking apple cider vinegar will not deplete your body while acidifying it. It has also been shown to help with weight loss and to promote the absorption of calcium and magnesium.

Over and over again it has been proven that the natural, whole food complexes that Mother Nature created are perfectly balanced to work with human physiology and to correct a vast number of disorders. Whole food supplements are the **only** supplements the body biochemically recognizes and can fully utilize.

Antioxidants—The Controversy

The debate over our need for antioxidants has been going on for some time. Often, those who advocate the need for antioxidants know nothing about whole food complexes. This is not surprising when most of the news about vitamins since the 1950s has been almost completely based on studies using the fractionated, crystalline-pure, synthetic chemicals.

The most widely touted antioxidants are vitamin E (d-alpha tocopherols), vitamin C (ascorbic acid), and beta-carotene. But taking antioxidants as stand-alone nutritional supplements means that we are " . . . ingesting fractions, isolated substances, not whole complexes. It would be like eating the peel of a banana without the banana, or like eating the shell of a nut without the nut meat." [52]

Few people realize that most commercial antioxidants are produced in pharmaceutical manufacturing plants. In 1992 *Time Magazine* reported that "Hoffman-LaRouche, for example, a huge pharmaceutical (drug) conglomerate, is building a plant in Freeport, Texas, to turn out 350 tons of synthetic beta-carotene, enough to supply a six milligram capsule daily to every American adult every year." [53]   No, there are not truckloads of carrots or any other natural foods going into that plant . . . except, possibly, in workers' lunchboxes.

Beta-carotene is only **one** carotenoid out of more than 600 that have been identified. Carotenoids give fruits and vegetables their colors. There are approximately 50 to 60 carotenes found in the typical American diet. To attribute a myriad of health benefits to a single carotene plays on the public's ignorance of the abundance of carotenoids already available in their foods.

There is much talk today about free radicals "attacking" human cells and weakening our immune systems. In deed they do. And, this is a natural oxidation process. When a molecule oxidizes, it goes from having an even to an odd number of electrons. (In stable molecules, electrons are always paired.) The free radical theory describes a destabilization reaction in which molecules steal or lose an electron, setting off a negative chain cascade.

However, as Judith De Cava points out, most honest scientists know that "every compound excreted by the body is in one form or another bound to oxygen for elimination." [54]

In simple terms, oxidation removes cellular waste and debris. It's nature's way of eliminating toxins from the body. So why are we making such a big deal about preventing a **necessary** process? To sell synthetic supplements, of course.

The Dark Side of Antioxidants

Most of the scientific research on synthesized antioxidants has been performed in test tubes or on microscope slides, not on humans. This has caused the researchers to overlook one tiny little detail: a person's ability to actually thrive on them.

The truth is too many synthetic antioxidants can cause fatigue and muscle weakness. Denham Harman, M.D., PhD., the "father" of the free radical theory of aging, was asked about the amounts of antioxidants he takes. Judith de Cava reports that "Dr. Harman listed an amazingly small amount compared to what many in the nutrition field are recommending: a maximum of 400 IU of 'vitamin E' (alpha-tocopherol) daily, 2,000 mg of 'vitamin C' (ascorbic acid) daily, and 25,000 IU of beta-carotene every other day. "I'd take more,' he said, 'but I can't afford to be fatigued.'" [55]

Toxic effects from large intakes of synthetic antioxidants have also been reported. This scenario sounds more like pharmaceutical drug side effects. It certainly doesn't jive with the image so highly promoted in ads and nutritional articles of antioxidants as being good for you—preventing disease and reversing the aging process.

In order to clearly understand what's going on here, let's review the pertinent facts about antioxidants:

- The process of oxidation that synthetic antioxidants are supposed to protect us from is a **natural** by-product of cellular combustion. Without it we would be dead.
- When taken in large doses synthetic antioxidants cause fatigue and muscular weakness.
- When taken in even larger doses these synthetic antioxidants are toxic.

The need for the public to take antioxidants has been promoted as a new "medical fact." Consequently, supplemental antioxidant consumption has become a standard practice among many nutritionally minded people. Unfortunately, the public is largely unaware of the mounting body of research that points to the dangers of taking antioxidants.

Fads, Trends, and Bold-Faced Lies

It is so easy for people to be taken in and manipulated to change their eating habits and/or their lifestyle in order to do something "healthy" for themselves. Before they know it, they're enrolled in a fad or a trend or a bold-faced lie. "Fad" is defined by *Webster's Dictionary* as "an exaggeratedly fussy attitude, especially about eating or not eating certain kinds of food."

Perhaps the most flagrant fad in our lifetime has been the low-fat diet craze. Only recently has science recognized the link between low-fat diets and the marked increase in diabetes, colds, fatigue, and depression. Over-refined grains loaded with synthetic supplements have significantly compromised our nation's health.

Webster's defines a trend as "a dominant movement revealed by a statistical process." American food consumption has been on an **unnatural** trend for nearly 100 years. Wall Street has come up with catchy slogans and slick marketing to cover up the dangers in our foods and our supplements. Because we believe the advertising, we have actually been altered as a culture: "we are not just unnatural—it is deeper. We are anti-natural." [56]

Bold-faced is defined by *Webster's* as "showing an impudent lack of shame." An impudent lack of shame is truly evident in those who proclaim the human body cannot tell the difference between synthetic vitamins and foods. Our current health crisis is proof that our bodies know the difference.

Why Do I Need Supplements If I'm Eating Well?

Vitamins are essential for human life. Needed only in small amounts in the diet, they regulate all metabolic processes, including growth, maintenance, energy production, reproduction and health. They also protect tissues against damage. Each

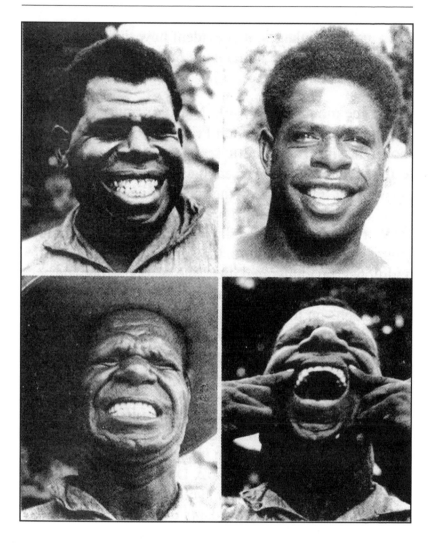

Natives on the islands of the Great Barrier Reef. The dental arches here reach a high degree of excellence.

Photos and captions by permission of the Price-Pottenger Foundation, California

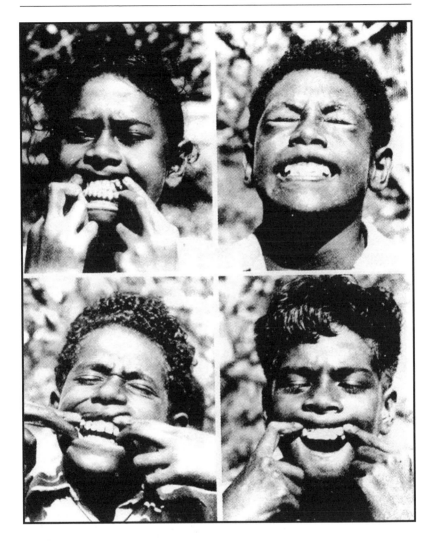

The contrast between the primitive and modernized natives in facial and dental arch form is as striking here as elsewhere. These young natives were born to parents who had adopted our modern foods of commerce. Note the narrowed faces and dental arches with pinched nostrils and crowding of the teeth. Their magnificent heredity could not protect them.

Photos and captions by permission of the Price-Pottenger Foundation, California

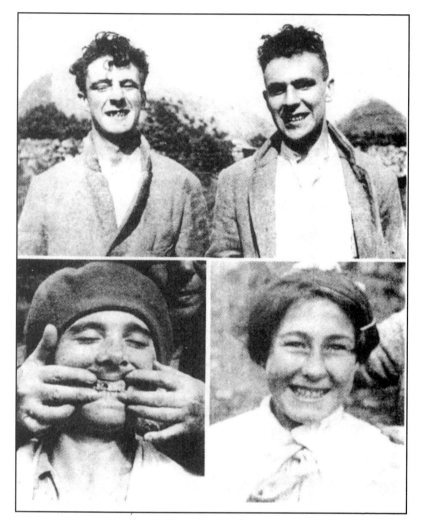

Above: Brothers, Isle of Harris. The younger at left uses modern food and has rampant tooth decay. Brother at right uses native food and has excellent teeth. Note narrowed face and arch of younger brother. Below left: typical rampant tooth decay, modernized Gaelic. Below right: typical excellent teeth of primitive Gaelic.

Photos and captions by permission of the Price-Pottenger Foundation, California

vitamin has its own special function in the body and cannot be replaced by anything else.

Vitamins are obtained from whole foods. Many people have likes and dislikes that keep them from eating green leafy vegetables such as kale, broccoli, Brussels sprouts and other foods necessary for good health. As a result, vitamin supplements are a must.

Let's face it, the commercial food industry has dominated America's eating habits for nearly 100 years. What most people don't realize is that it has taken a cumulative toll on us, weakening us from generation to generation. From the 1930s onward, the nutritional deficiencies these foods created began to **alter our genes!** Dr. Royal Lee was one of the first to recognize that over-processed foods caused " . . . the previously unanticipated phenomenon of many genetically transmitted conditions, because they originated in deficiency and poisoning patterns of forbearers." [57]

The monumental work of Dr. Weston Price, D.D.S., *Nutrition and Physical Degeneration,* captured the destruction of the health of primitive peoples around the world as soon as they began eating the foods the white man introduced: white flour products, polished rice, jams, marmalades, vegetable oils, canned meats and vegetables, confections and fruits. "As soon as parents began to eat what Dr. Price called '*the foods of commerce*,' they passed along inferior genetic traits to the very next generation of offspring." [58] Their faces changed shape, their immunity was lost, and childbearing became painful and difficult. (See illustrations.)

First published in 1945, Dr. Price's book was initially required reading in medical and dental schools and also in anthropology classes at Harvard University. Within a couple of years this revealing book was pulled from the schools' library shelves and fell into obscurity. It was a wakeup call then and is even more of a wakeup call today. How many generations are we into this altered genetic transmission?

Dr. Price took careful chemical analysis of all the foods the indigenous peoples ate and compared them with American foods in the 1930s. At that time he estimated the primitives ate from 4 to 10 times more vitamins and minerals every day than Americans did. This means that the processed and refined American diet was deficient to the tune of between 1,500 and 3,650 nutrients in a single year.

The result? We are not as strong as our ancestors. We are somewhere in the second, third, fourth or fifth generation in this over-processed and ruined diet transmission. We are in need of as much nutritional rebuilding as we can possibly get. To continue to consume synthetic vitamins to build up a body already weakened by depleted foods and synthetic vitamins simply does not work. (More of nothing does not equal more of anything.)

With such a heavy loss of nutrients, no wonder so many people have infertility problems today. In 1952 Dr. Lee wrote, "I could write volumes on how synthetic vitamins, like thiamine, castrate the descendants of the victim who uses even as much as double the daily requirements." [59]

A study was done by Dr. Barnett Sure (*J. Nutr.,* August 1939) on two groups of pigs; one group was fed twice the daily requirements of synthetic B vitamin, and the other group the same amount of natural B vitamin. What he found was that "ALL of the first generation offspring from the pigs fed the synthetic vitamin were STERILE....Obviously, synthetic B is NOT A NUTRIENT, it is a genetic poison that damages the chromosome packages responsible for transmitting sexual characteristics from the parent to the offspring." [60]

Humans, unlike pigs, take more than one generation to manifest genetic damage of this magnitude. A 1981 report from the University of Florida stated that the American male sperm count in 1929 was approximately 100 million sperm cells per milliliter of semen. By 1973 the sperm count had dropped to 60 million. Only seven years later, in 1980, the count had dropped to 20 million.

What happened here? Richard P. Murray, D.C. suggests the answer "could very well lie in the historical use of synthetic B and other counterfeit nutrients....Since World War II the American people, and people of other countries as well, have had a daily ration of a genetic poison in most of the bread, flour products, cereals and other food items that are forced by law, to enrich with the only cost-feasible enricher: synthetic vitamins."[61] (A dead food + a dead vitamin could = a recipe for disaster.)

A Word About Standard Process

In 1929 Dr. Lee developed his first supplement, which he named Catalyn® because the whole food vitamins, minerals and enzymes it contained acted as organic catalysts. These catalysts speeded up metabolic processes by providing people with what was lacking in their diets. People noticed a marked increase in both their vitality and resistance to infection when taking it.

Dr. Lee's strategy for marketing Catalyn was to have it distributed through health professionals so that people could be taken care of at the very onset of their condition. In order to do so, he had to compile case studies and present them to the health care providers. As more and more people with extreme health conditions were introduced to Catalyn and experienced remarkable results, news spread quickly throughout the United States. Dr. Lee then began developing branch offices to service health professionals across the country.

With Catalyn's remarkable success, Dr. Lee began researching other whole food supplement products, including products that contained a whole vitamin complex, his Cataplex® series of products. For his Cataplex E he tapped the richest food source he had discovered: the whole pea vine plant.

From the very beginning, Dr. Lee purchased raw materials for his supplements that were pesticide free. In order to have more control over quality, he ended up purchasing his own farmland.

Dr. Lee picked the farm's location in Wisconsin specifically for its abundance of glacier-deposited minerals. Over the years, the size of Standard Process organic farms has grown to over 1,000 acres. In its renowned, thick black topsoil, today Standard Process grows hundreds of thousands of pounds of crops each year for use in their supplements. These crops include alfalfa, beets, buckwheat, Spanish black radish, pea vine, Brussels sprouts, carrots, buckwheat, and oats.

Since Dr. Royal Lee believed that we, as humans, need the nutrition from both plants *and* animals for optimum health, he began investigating how to extract nutrients from animal organs and tissues to use in his products. In the 1940s he was finally able to derive tissue extracts from specific organs and glands known as cell determinants, which he called Protomorphogens™. These extracts were particularly important in both supporting and helping to restore normal cell function. Throughout the 1950s he developed over 20 specific Protomorphogen products.

Dr. Lee's research also led him to the development of what he called the Cytosol™ extract. This extract contained all of the cellular factors that are the biochemical building blocks essential to cellular metabolism. Today there are six specific Cytosol products, but many of the Standard Process products contain either or both of the Protomorphogen and Cytosol extracts along with raw nutrient-rich plant materials.

When we take these potent Standard Process supplements, we are given something really special—a chance to "catch up" for lost time nutritionally. What this really means is best illustrated by the following quote from Dr. Bruce West, whose well-known newsletter, *Health Alert*, has helped thousands of people on the road to health: "If you had a heart problem with high blood fats and poor digestion, my best R_x would be some powerful dietary changes. For starters, if this was feasible, I would like to see you consume daily: a pound of raw, organic liver: a couple of buckets of organic wheat germ and high-selenium yeast; a small wheelbarrow full of organic beets and beet tops; gallons of freshly squeezed vegetable juices; and plenty of raw, fresh-pressed organic oils, such as flax seed oil. Naturally, this is impossible. So, instead, we use supplements which are condensed from these foods and other nutrients." [62]

For making all these wonderful contributions to the health of humanity, Dr. Lee was continually persecuted and harassed by the FDA. He distributed a massive amount of product literature in which he contended that illnesses, such as functional heart problems, and degenerative diseases, such as arthritis, could be traced to a lack of vitamins and other necessary food factors in the American diet. The FDA reviewed this literature and concluded that it was inconsistent with what they contended was the current consensus of medical opinion. Therefore, it was branded "false and misleading" and Dr. Lee was fined and put on three years' probation.

Finally, he submitted to signing a Consent Decree with the FDA that allowed them to destroy all research they deemed to be "misleading" from the Standard Process headquarters. Reports have it that large fires in barrels burned for nearly a month. It's hard to believe that this happened in the United States in the early 1960s—instead of in Nazi Germany in 1939.

The Work in Nutrition Has Already Been Done

Every time a new micronutrient is discovered, it's discovered in foods. And, every time these discoveries are made, Catalyn is analyzed to see if it contains it. And it always does. Why? Because Catalyn was designed by drawing on a number of whole foods to contain every nutrient needed to support a human being's biochemistry. Dr. Lee believed that whole foods are really a blend of untold numbers, types, and variations of nutrient complexes.

What does this tell us? That Mother Nature has already done all the work in nutrition! Nature is the chemist, and all that a biochemist can do is to unlock **the already existing relation-**

ships within and among all of these micronutrient factors, split them up, identify them, and test them to see what happens when a laboratory animal goes without them.

This is really what is happening when you hear about a new "discovery." Co-enzyme Q-10, co-enzyme PQQ, synthetic antioxidants (like beta-carotene and pycnogenols), selenium and phytochemicals are all perfect examples of "discoveries" that are already present in whole foods. When you purchase a bottle of d-alpha tocopherol vitamin E capsules, a bottle of selenium, and a bottle of co-enzyme Q10, what you actually have are isolated, synthetic parts of the vitamin E complex that are all dead and inert. Not only that, but there are many other components that you are simply not getting, and it is impossible to get the correct dosage of even one component!

A Sobering Word

J.I. Rodale, the American naturalist, made this wise statement in his classic work *The Complete Book of Food and Nutrition*: "We must take vitamins if we wish to be healthy and the nation as a whole must do it, or God alone knows what will happen to the second or third generations coming up—generations inheriting weaknesses passed on to them by us, generations which few will live to see unless we augment our diet with vitamins and minerals. And, as parting advice, don't take coal tar (synthetic) vitamins. Examine every bottle. Be sure that the vitamins you take are extracted from food. Scientific research proves that this is best." [63]

It couldn't have been said any better. Remember, thiamine HCl and thiamine mononitrate both come from coal tar and are in all commercial breads. Synthetic vitamin B_{12} comes from activated sewage sludge, vitamin E from refined and heated oils, and synthetic vitamin D is concocted from irradiated oil.

Bon Appetit!

If the members of the American Medical establishment were to have a collective find-yourself-naked-in-Times-Square-nightmare, this might be it. They spend 30 years ridiculing Robert Atkins…accusing the Manhattan doctor of quackery and fraud, only to discover that the unrepentant Atkins was right all along. Or maybe it's this: They find that their very own dietary recommendations—eat less fat and more carbohydrates—are the cause of the rampaging epidemic of obesity in America. Or, just possibly this: They find out both of the above are true."

Gary Taubes
"What If It's Been A Big Fat Lie?"
New York Times Magazine, July 7, 2002

3/ Fats, Proteins, Carbohydrates and Your Health

With much of our food supply over processed and synthetic vitamins added to everything, what else could be done to ruin our health? Well, we could be encouraged to eat a **low-fat diet** (often low in protein and high in carbohydrate as well), thus ensuring that we ingest more over refined foods and create blood sugar problems that can really wreak havoc with our metabolism and our health.

A Historical Perspective

At the turn of the 20th Century Americans were heavy meat eaters and some of the healthiest people in the world. With rapid industrial and economic development came some significant changes. Food historian Harvey Levenstein reports in his epic book, *Revolution at the Table: The Transformation of the American Diet*, that the substitution of one kind of food for another was perhaps the most dramatic of these changes.

Those most successful at creating this substitution were "the entrepreneurs of the breakfast food industry who almost single-handedly destroyed the traditional American breakfast. . . . The breakfast food manufacturers managed to promote…the replacement of the traditional slabs of meat with various forms of highly processed grain." [64]

Other food processors were greatly influenced by the marketing techniques of these early cereal manufacturers. "The rise of Kellogg's 'Corn Flakes' and Post's 'Grape-Nuts' and 'Toasties,' which led the way, held important lessons for other food processors. First, there was the link to health. . . . Post, a master of the dubious health claim whose genius lay in slogans that implied everything but promised nothing, marketed his cereal as a 'brain food' which was also likely to cure consumption, malaria, and loose teeth. Second, of course, there was convenience. . . . Third, there was hygiene. . . . The neatly packaged cereals promised absolute cleanliness and, presumably, germ-free food." [65]

What followed in the wake of this first wave of food substitution were all the signs of physical degeneration that Dr. Weston Price's study proved would happen. When Dr. Price looked up the statistics from the Department of Health for New York City from 1907 to 1936, the records showed a 60% increase in heart disease and a 90% increase in cancer during that time period! Food substitution was clearly taking its toll.

The American Diet Today

Nearly a century later, what does the typical American eat? The Center for Disease Control's National Center for Health Statistics published data in 1983 detailing the food consumption patterns of Americans. "What would you guess as the number-one food consumed by the most Americans? White bread, rolls, and crackers—almost pure carbohydrate. How about number two? Doughnuts, cookies, and cake—more carbohydrate and fat. Number three, alcoholic beverages. All in all, of the top twenty foods Americans eat, eleven are virtually pure carbohydrate, four are a combination of carbohydrate and protein, and only five are pure protein or a combination of protein and fat. . . . *89 percent of the American diet is fat and carbohydrate.*" [66] If we look around us and see what people are eating today, these statistics have only gotten worse.

This kind of food consumption is literally a recipe for disaster. The growing number of diabetics and the alarming rise in obesity, especially in children, tell us that the food we are putting in our mouths is promoting disease, not health. These numbers also demonstrate how the low fat diet has been embraced by our nation.

How Did It Happen?

Gary Taubes, a journalist who writes for the journal *Science*, traces the evolution of the low-fat diet through a jungle of mishaps: scientific "leaps of faith," political agendas, media frenzies, and food industry concoctions. The bottom line is that we should think twice about following the government's Food Guide Pyramid. In fact, we really should think twice (or more) about how our health is being negatively affected by orthodox medicine and mainstream "nutritional science."

At first the low-fat diet concept seemed to make sense. It claimed that the saturated fat found in meat and dairy products elevates cholesterol levels, which are then supposed to clog our arteries (atherosclerosis) and cause a heart attack. Fat came to be seen as the arch-villain, and over the years different waves of public anxiety about fat have rolled across the land, changing our eating habits but not improving our health.

One of the early anxiety waves held that dietary fat caused cancer. This proposition was thought to be incontrovertible in the late 1970s. "Fifteen years and hundreds of millions of dollars later, a . . . massive expert report by the World Cancer Research Fund and the American Institute for Cancer Research could find neither 'convincing' nor even 'probable' reason to believe that dietary fat caused cancer." [67]

Then along came the theory that cutting dietary fat caused weight loss. Remember being told over and over that carbohydrates and protein have 4 calories per gram and fat has 9 calories, so cutting fat will cut pounds? This made perfect sense—or so we thought. "Considerable data, however, now suggest other wise. The results of well controlled clinical trials are consistent: People on low-fat diets initially lose a couple of kilograms, as they would on any diet, and then the weight tends to return." [68]

And guess what? Since the 1970s Americans actually have cut their fat consumption, and obesity has surged upward. Today one in four Americans is considered obese and the number of people who are diagnosed with Type 2 diabetes is exploding.

The Link with Heart Disease

The link between dietary fat consumption and heart disease has been tangled up in the cholesterol-lowering issue since 1984 when the administrators of the $140 million Lipid Research Clinics (LRC) Coronary Primary Prevention Trial decided to jump into the dietary fat debate.

This lipid research trial was **not** a diet trial. It was a drug trial, testing to see if the medication cholestyramine could reduce heart disease by lowering cholesterol levels. The outcome of the seven-year study was released in 1984 and the results were marginal, if not pathetic: the probability of dying from a heart attack was reduced from 2.0% to 1.6%. (Whoopee!)

Not to be stopped by such a paltry improvement with cholestyramine, Basil Rifkind from the National Heart, Lung, and Blood Institute (NHLBI) and his colleagues "concluded, without the benefit of dietary data, that cholestyramine's benefits could be extended to diet as well . . . They felt they could never actually demonstrate that low-fat diets prolonged lives—that would be too expensive—but now they had established a fundamental link in the causal chain, from lower cholesterol levels to cardiovascular health. With that, they could take the leap of faith from cholesterol-lowering drugs and health to cholesterol-lowering diet and health." [69]

The media then pushed the low-fat message, boosting the massive health campaign that was launched. *Time Magazine* reported "the LRC findings under the headline, 'Sorry, It's True. Cholesterol really is a killer.' The article about a drug trial began: 'No whole milk. No butter. No fatty meats . . .' *Time* followed up 3 months later with a cover story: 'And Cholesterol and Now the Bad News . . .' the cover photo was a frowning face: a breakfast plate with two fried eggs as the eyes and a bacon strip for the mouth. Rifkind was quoted as saying that their results 'strongly indicate that the more you lower cholesterol and fat in your diet, the more you reduce your risk of heart disease,' a statement that still lacked direct scientific support." [70]

The Government and the Food Industry Step In

A few years before this entirely unscientific leap of faith, Senator George McGovern's bipartisan Select Committee on Nutrition and Human Needs had listened to a meager two days of testimony on diet and disease in July 1976. From these two days emerged the document, "Dietary Goals for the United States," recommending that Americans cut their fat intake to 30% of the calories they consumed and cut consumption of saturated fat to 10%. (McGovern and his wife had both signed on to participate in no-fat diet guru Nathan Pritikin's diet and exercise plan. Although McGovern did quit the program early, Pritikin was a major influence on his thinking.)

Seven years later the USDA turned McGovern's recommendations into public policy with the release of the revised Food Guide Pyramid that had pictures of pasta, rice and bread at the base of the pyramid. (6-11 servings were suggested.) One of the most amazing observations we can make is the disparity between the **whole** grains recommended in the "Dietary Goals" and the USDA Food Pyramid and the over processed foods that have always filled our supermarket shelves.

To get people to blame themselves and not the government for this contradictory input into the American psyche, well-intentioned government officials are portrayed as frustrated because Americans are eating doughnuts, white bread, and cake instead of the suggested whole grain foods, fruit, vegetables and legumes. Hmm . . . could this be economics at work?

Alan Stone, a staff director for McGovern's Senate committee told Taubes that he had an inkling of how the food industry would respond to the new "Dietary Goals" back when the hearings were first held. "An economist pulled him aside, he said, and gave him a lesson in market disincentives to healthy eating: 'He said if you create a new market with a brand-new manufactured food, give it a brand-new fancy name, put a big advertising budget behind it, you can have a market all to yourself and force your competitors to catch up. You can't do that with fruits and vegetables. It's harder to differentiate an apple from an apple." [71]

To date, over 15,000 low-fat foods have been created to "meet the needs" of the public to eat the low-fat way. But in order to create low-fat foods that tasted good enough to eat, adding more sugar made up for the loss of taste that went with the fat; and products that never had any fat to begin with, like Big Gulps and Coca Cola, advertised themselves as "100 percent fat free."

Was All This REALLY Necessary?

How could such an erroneous scientific concept get started in the first place? Historically, fear of fat really took off after World War II when an epidemic of coronary heart disease swept the country. In the words of biochemist Ancel Keys at the University of Minnesota, "Middle-aged men, seemingly healthy, were dropping dead." [72]   Heart Disease was quickly labeled "the

If you're surprised by the information you've read in this book and you're beginning to re-think issues surrounding your health, there is SO much more I've discovered I want you to know about. In fact, although you're not aware of this yet, just by reading *Going Back to The Basics of Human Health* you have entered the realms of . . .

THE PERFECT CRIME!
(A unique approach to understanding your health issues)

Tear out this form, pay a visit to www.theperfectcrime.com and sign up for my Investigative Health Reports.

Your journey has just begun!

silent killer," and it was Dr. Keys who first suggested that the culprit was fat.

But what else was happening after World War II that Dr. Keys and many others totally ignored? Harvey Levenstein calls this period in America's food history "The Golden Age of Food Processing." All of the technology that had been used for the manufacturing of C-rations was redirected into mass-producing new foods that required the creation of hundreds of food additives. Soon, large-scale equipment replaced human handling with continuous operations where automatic equipment (robots) now sucked, dumped, filtered, mixed, extruded, fermented, cooled, fried, drained, and packaged foods.

And the supermarket was born. "Better Living Through Chemistry" was the industry motto. Home economists couldn't be enthusiastic enough. Women's magazines happily carried articles extolling how "the day is coming when a woman can buy a boiled dinner and carry it home in her purse…when you'll serve the girls a bridge luncheon of dehydrated meat and potatoes with powdered potatoes and powdered onions, a dehydrated cabbage salad, and custard made with powdered eggs and powdered milk for dessert." [73]

And the scientists didn't notice? If it had not been for one lone congressman who parlayed some political debts into permission to head a commission to investigate the increased use of chemicals in foods, we would know very little about what was going on inside the food industry at all—even today.

The Delaney Hearings

The lone congressman was James Delaney from Brooklyn and the hearings he headed in 1951 and 1952 were known as the hearings on "Chemicals in Food Products." At first, scientists with the food and chemical industries actually refused to justify their practices. These industries were not used to **any** scrutiny, since they felt adequately protected by the Nutrition Foundation they had set up in 1941 to head off any such questioning.

But Delaney got his way and, 1,460 pages of testimony later, many unsettling facts had come out. The first fact was that the food industry policed itself. Only after an additive entered interstate commerce could the FDA then determine if it was poisonous. And if the FDA did deem an additive to be poisonous it took several years to get it pulled from the marketplace.

The second discovery was that **no** scientific body was qualified to determine whether or not a food is harmful. (Dr. Wiley's Bureau of Chemistry was the only authority that had been written into law, and it was gone.) The food industry was just too busy developing ingredients, putting them into foods and getting these foods to market to take the time to test an ingredient for safety.

All negative information presented at the hearings about the chemicals in foods came from independent studies. One found that certain bread softeners caused kidney stones and diarrhea in rats. A ten-year study done by Dr. Clive McCoy, professor of nutrition at Cornell University, reported that when teeth were placed in the same phosphoric acid found in cola drinks, they softened and began to dissolve. (This is especially interesting in light of the fact that the only criticism we ever hear about soft drinks today is that they contain too much sugar.)

The final outcome of the Delaney Hearings was the determination that the public was entitled to greater protection with respect to the foods they consumed and that no such existing legislation gave the public this protection. In 1958 Congress passed the Delaney Amendment. It suggested that maybe food processors should prove that their chemicals were safe for humans. (But they didn't have to if they didn't want to.) One clause (the one we have heard so much about over the years) forbade the use of any substance that caused cancer in rats. The only safe dose is zero.

To this day there has been absolutely no change to what was discovered in the Delaney Hearings. Furthermore, the zero risk turned into such a nightmare for the food industry that they finally had it done away with in the "Food Quality Protection Act of 1996."

At the time of the Delaney Hearings, there were 704 chemicals in foods. In 1984 Ruth Winter's *A Consumer's Dictionary of Food Additives* covered over 8,000 additives used in our foods. Her updated edition in 2004 covers over 12,000 additives! Today, even if legislation were passed calling for removal of a pesticide, the pesticide companies have five years to **begin** to pull the designated pesticide from the marketplace. After that, they have up to seven years to show that this pesticide isn't dangerous to our food supply.

Getting to the Point

Let's get back to fat. How did fat get to be blamed as the cause of all the heart attacks after World War II when there were so many other obvious places to look? One might think that the sheer numbers of new chemicals machined into the food supply would catch the interest of a scientist or two. But, what about the question of nutrient-loss in the foods even **before** the robots got hold of them? Could this be at the root of the heart attacks?

Dr. Royal Lee pointed out in a 1946 talk to naturopaths that "It has been found by experiment that if cattle are fed on grain from which the germ has been removed, they will continue to gain in weight, and appear to remain in perfect health. But, before many months they begin to drop dead from heart failure. There is no warning in their behavior, no apparent change in their condition of health. . . . Since practically all the cereal products found in human diets are degerminated at the factory to keep out bug infestation, it is quite clear to any rational person why the incidence of heart disease has increased progressively with the increase in the sale of such cereal products." [74]

Lee certainly explained why heart disease was labeled the "silent killer." But we need to remember that Dr. Lee's work was branded "false and misleading" by the FDA because it was inconsistent with the current consensus of medical opinion.

Pointing out the dangers of removing the nutrient-rich germ of grains from foods was not consistent with the consensus of medical opinion, but pointing to fat as the arch-villain was. We can also see from the rise (and now falling) concept of the low-fat diet that the "consensus" of medical opinion was not really a consensus.   Maverick doctors—Atkins, Flatt and Blackburn among them—had tested diets containing plenty of fat from the 1970s on with great success. Atkins was the one openly called a quack.

Today, with the public led to consume far more refined carbohydrates than ever before, the health of our nation is being ruined. Americans with elevated blood pressure, cholesterol and blood sugar levels swamp our health care system today.

What Happens When We Consume A Lot Of Carbs?

When we consume carbohydrates, we are really consuming sugar . . . in a different form. Bite into a piece of bread and hold it in your mouth for moments without chewing it. You will notice that it tastes sweet. This is because all carbohydrates are composed of sugar (glucose) molecules bonded together chemically. Your body's digestive process breaks these chemical bonds and releases sugar molecules into the blood stream.

At that point, your blood sugar will begin to climb and your pancreas will secrete the hormone insulin into the bloodstream. "The insulin travels to the liver and to the muscle cells, telling them to take glucose from the bloodstream and store it. . . . As insulin levels increase, blood-glucose levels begin to fall. Once blood glucose falls below a critical level, the brain, which needs glucose to function, begins to call out for more glucose. If the brain doesn't get the glucose it wants, it starts tuning out. Medically, this glucose shortage is known as hypoglycemia or low blood sugar. When it happens to adults, it produces mental fatigue. That's why when you eat a big pasta meal at noon by three o'clock you can barely keep your eyes open." [75]

Sound familiar?

Our Bodies' Complexity

When we hear the word *hormone* we usually think of the sex hormones estrogen and testosterone, but in truth hormones regulate every single metabolic function. They are really the "micro-messengers" that form the communication system in our bodies. Hormones usually come in pairs, each hormone in the pair having the opposite physiological effect from the other.

For example, the hormone insulin is responsible for bringing blood sugar levels down when they are too high, and its paired hormone glucagon increases blood sugar levels. Insulin also causes our metabolism to store food energy for later. Glucagon allows our bodies to burn our stored fat for energy.

These functions of storing and burning fat are active to some degree all the time. The question is, which energy pathway dominates? Are we mainly storing or mainly burning fat for energy? It is important to note that fat in the bloodstream comes from three sources: fat consumed in the diet, fat made from excess carbohydrates and protein in the diet, and fat liberated from storage in the fat cells.

It is an unappreciated fact that our bodies make fat from dietary carbohydrate—low fat cookies and potato chips include. So much for the fallacy of low-fat foods!

Excess Insulin and Obesity

Eating a high-carbohydrate diet keeps the pancreas secreting insulin in order to bring blood sugar levels down. But when the pancreas has to work all the time and insulin levels remain high, the body is constantly in a fat storage mode. Glucagon doesn't have a chance to come in and start burning up the stored fat, which can certainly explain why obese people who have attempted dieting over and over again on low-fat diets have failed.

But excess insulin levels do more than make people fat. Drs. Michael R. Eades and Mary Dan Eades explain in their book, *Protein Power*, that excess insulin levels are the hidden cause behind high blood pressure, high blood cholesterol and triglyceride levels, adult-onset diabetes, and heart disease.

How? In the case of high blood pressure, insulin is working behind the scenes, actually forcing the kidneys to retain sodium, resulting in fluid retention. "As the body retains more fluid and the blood volume increases, the blood pressure begins to rise and in due course reach dangerous levels, requiring treatment." [76] This is the reason that diuretics work so well to control high blood pressure.

Excessive amounts of insulin also increase the thickness of the arterial walls, making them less elastic and narrower, which drives blood pressure up. Ultimately, the Drs. Eades make a compelling case: insulin stimulates the adrenals to constrict blood vessels, increasing the heart rate and raising blood pressure.

What usually happens when you go to your doctor for a regular checkup and find that your cholesterol level and blood pressure are too high? You leave the office with instructions to go on a low-fat diet and return to the office for a recheck in a month or so. "With this protein and fat restriction, the only food component left in the diet is carbohydrate, which by default results in your eating a high-carbohydrate, low-protein diet—the very diet that maximizes insulin production." [77]

You revisit the doctor's office a month later and the doctor finds that your cholesterol levels are down slightly, though not in the normal range and your blood pressure levels are the same or a little higher. This time you leave the doctor's office with a more rigid diet, a prescription for a high blood pressure medicine and another for a cholesterol-lowering medicine.

When you next return for your follow-up visit with your doctor, "your doctor finds that your blood pressure level has fallen into the normal range. You are relieved and happy, and the drug companies are ecstatic: they have just signed you on as a new customer . . . for life." [78]

WARNING: The Drs. Eades found that a high protein/low carbohydrate diet was so effective in lowering blood pressure that their patients who were on medication to lower their blood pressure felt dizzy and faint within a few days and had to be taken off their medication very quickly. Do not attempt this diet if you are on medication to lower your blood pressure without being under the care of a physician.

Excess Insulin and Cholesterol

Worrying about cholesterol levels has sent people by the droves into their doctors' offices, and tinkering with cholesterol levels has become big business. The Drs. Eades point out, "whenever mass paranoia starts to brew, a legion rises up ready to exploit it. The food processing industry and their advertisers now emblazon the containers of edibles as diverse as soft drinks and cornflakes with the superfluous statement 'contains no cholesterol.' Cholesterol angst is not lost on the various governmental and private research funding bodies responsible for underwriting all kinds of medical research. These groups disburse hundreds of millions of dollars to eager research labs throughout the world, allowing them to pursue the secrets of cholesterol in ever-more intricate studies." [79]

Cholesterol, as the Drs. Eades explain, is essential for life. Only 7% of the body's cholesterol is found in the blood. "The bulk of the cholesterol in your body, the other 93% is located in every cell of the body, where its unique waxy, soapy consistency provides the cell membranes with their structural integrity and regulates the flow of nutrients into, and waste products out of, the cells." [80]

Cholesterol is the building block for all hormones and the major component of liver bile. Your brain and nerves require cholesterol for normal electrical transmission. Some cholesterol comes from food, but the body itself produces 80%, mostly by the liver.

The main point here is that our cholesterol levels are actually regulated **inside** the trillions of cells that make up our bodies. If a cell needs more cholesterol, it sends LDL (low-density lipoprotein) receptors to the surface in order to snatch cholesterol from the blood. LDL, although often depicted as the Bad Guy in the cholesterol drama, is the component of cholesterol that carries it to the cells. HDL, or high-density lipoprotein, gathers cholesterol from the tissues and carries it back to the liver to be disposed of. The flow one way or another is what medical researchers have used to quantify risk for heart disease.

Excess insulin in the blood causes LDL levels to rise. Excess carbohydrates cause excess insulin.

Excess Insulin and Diabetes

Today diabetes is widespread. We all know someone who has been diagnosed with it. More and more and more children are being diagnosed with it. The Drs. Eades trace this growing problem back to the huge consumption of sugary foods and carbohydrates that turn into sugar. A kid who consumes soft drinks, candy bars, cookies and ice cream every day could end up consuming over two cups of pure sugar a day.

At this rate of consumption the blood sugar levels stay high all the time. The pancreas is constantly working. At some point the metabolic gears begin to slip, and the cells in the body become insulin resistant. This means that the receptors inside the cells no longer respond adequately to insulin, and the pancreatic beta cells that produce the insulin have to put out ever-increasing amounts of insulin. "Under constant overstimulation by the excess glucose the beta cells may finally give up and cease producing insulin altogether—a condition called *beta cell fatigue* or *beta cell burnout*. . . . High blood sugar or hyperglycemia then becomes not only a manifestation of diabetes but a self-perpetuating cause of the disorder as well."[81]

Eric M. Bost, Under Secretary of Food, Nutrition and Consumer Services, testified in 2004 "Diabetes has increased by

49% in the past 10 years, reflecting strong correlation with obesity. . . . It is increasingly diagnosed in children and adolescents; 1 in 3 persons born in 2000 will develop diabetes if there is no change in current health habits. . . . Recent trends among children are alarming: in the past 20 years, the percentage of children who are overweight has doubled and the percentage of adolescents who are overweight has more than tripled. If we do not stem this tide, many children in this generation will not outlive their parents."[82] The result of excess insulin gone rampant.

Excess Insulin and Heart Disease

"A heart attack occurs when, for whatever reason, the blood flow to an area of the heart is cut off or severely diminished"[83]
The process starts when LDL particles migrate into the walls of the coronary arteries, setting off an inflammatory process that leads to the buildup of plaque. By sustaining high levels of insulin in the blood, low-fat, high carbohydrate diets play an integral part in the plaque-building process.

Dr. John Abramson, author of *Overdosed America: The Broken Promise of American Medicine*, says that most heart attacks are not caused by the gradual buildup of plaque, but are the result of a small area of this plaque becoming eroded on its surface and breaking open. "This causes the tiny platelets circulating in the blood to become sticky and form a small blood clot, or thrombus, on the top of the plaque. Without any warning, thrombus formation can quickly and completely obstruct the flow of blood through a coronary artery, causing a heart attack."[84]

Although no one knows for sure what causes the plaque to break open, we do know that excess insulin aggravates the creation and buildup of plaque—and many other processes we don't want going on in our bodies. Making the necessary dietary changes to keep insulin under control is one of the best things you can do for your health and your well-being.

Controlling Insulin with Diet

The only way to truly control insulin is with diet, and unless we understand the special role of the eicosanoids, we ignore the vital role that good fats play in maintaining our health. MIT researcher Barry Sears first introduced us to eicosanoids in 1995. Sears explained that there are almost 100 powerful eicosanoids in the body. "Mysterious and fleeting but all-powerful, eicosanoids are made by every living cell in the human body. They're the molecular glue that holds the human body together." [85]

There are "good" eicosanoids, such as the ones that help us sleep well, keep our immune system up and decrease pain. There are also the "bad" eicosanoids, the ones that cause us to sleep poorly, give us headaches and cause the formation of tumors. Both good and bad eicosanoids are produced from linoleic acid, which is present in all foods.

The key to health is to get sufficient linoleic acid into the system and do what it takes to shift the balance toward the good side of the eicosanoid equation. In order to speed up the body's gatekeeper, the *delta 6-desaturase enzyme*, we need to eat plenty of protein. Factors that slow this gatekeeper down are aging, stress, disease, trans fats and high-carbohydrate diets.

Obviously, there is not too much we can do about aging. Our fast-paced American way of life makes stress a common factor in almost everyone's life. And no matter how hard we try, we still get the occasional cold or flu.

We need to take control of our health where we can and diet is the key. Diet is the main way for all of us to exercise control over our health and create a sense of well-being. By eating high protein meals (and snacks), adding good unrefined oils to our diets, avoiding trans fats and cutting down on carbohydrates we can do a lot to cut down on excess insulin, produce good eicosanoids and experience good health.

"As I see it, I have spent about two percent
of my life developing new and useful products. The other
ninety-eight percent of my time has been occupied with a
constant battle with someone to make him believe the facts on
which my work is based."

Dr. Royal Lee

4/ Our Health

What is "good health?" Sadly, we really don't know anymore.

The World Health Organization defines health as a "state of complete physical, mental, and social well-being and not merely the absence of disease or infirmity." [86] Dr. Francis Pottenger defined health as the result of an optimal diet, "one which provides man with the nutrients essential to regenerate his body cells; to enable him to mature regularly as determined by his normal [skeletal], physical, and mental characteristics; to resist disease; to reproduce his kind [in succeeding generations]; and to enable him to produce a livelihood for his family." [87]

Let's just start by taking an informal survey of our American health profile by noticing people's appearance. Every day you and I see people with pasty, sallow complexions—yellow, gray, or sometimes white. We see pasty complexions so often that it never occurs to us these folks have poor blood quality or that something else is wrong. "That's just the way they look . . ."

There is hardly a grocery store, fast food chain, post office or bank you can enter without seeing someone with a wrist immobilized in a brace for carpel-tunnel syndrome. Repetitive work is blamed for this. Never does it occur to us that human ligaments are weakened by insufficient protein, vitamin C complex, calcium and manganese.

Today children are born with all kinds of abnormalities. Dr. Weston Price was adamant that to produce normal healthy babies, the parents must be fed optimal nutrition **before conception** and during pregnancy. Ubiquitous trans fats block nutrients from being utilized by the human body—in this case, blocking nutrients from getting to the fetus. When consumed by pregnant women, trans fats lead to low birth weight in newborns: the U.S. is 74th in the world in infant mortality due to low birth weight.

Childhood asthma is on the rise, and few parents realize that the trans fats in the breads, cookies, cakes, and crackers their children consume on a daily basis can precipitate it. Many children are frequently sick, yet few parents realize that the high fructose corn syrup in the sodas and juices their children consume actually weaken their immune systems. While the consumption of pizza and other fast foods is rampant in our schools nearly 6 million children have been diagnosed and put on amphetamines for ADHD—a condition that has been consistently tied to the wooziness of hypoglycemia, the result of eating too many carbohydrates.

Other health problems such as bruising easily, bleeding gums, stretch marks, painful joints, popping or cracking of the joints and slipped discs are just accepted as "normal wear and tear" on the body. But these are all signs of subclinical scurvy, a vitamin C complex deficiency.

Impaired wound healing is a common phenomenon. Hair loss, dry skin, and eczema are also common complaints. These conditions are often due to a Vitamin F or fatty-acid deficiency, along with a toxic bowel. Most people are unaware that partially hydrogenated oils (trans fats) block the good fatty acids from entering the cells in our bodies. With this comes a loss of calcium assimilation and persistent, high blood sugar levels because insulin can't get into the cells either.

We rationalize all this and more and keep on moving—tiredly. Fatigue has become such a widespread symptom that we even have a medical name for it: Chronic Fatigue Syndrome.

Look in the Mirror

One of the most common nutritional deficiencies in America today is a vitamin B complex deficiency (BCD). Here are some symptoms of BCD: indigestion; weakness and fatigue; dizziness; forgetfulness; uneasiness; rage; anxiety; irregular heart beat; depression: mental confusion: insomnia; and craving for sweets.

The tendency to cry for no reason at all is a red flag for vitamin B complex deficiency; but the classic symptom of BCD is the constant feeling that something dreadful is about to happen. There are so many emotional components to nutritional deficiencies, especially of the B vitamin complex. Yet many people, failing to recognize the physical deficiency, believe that something is psychologically wrong with them. Those astute enough to realize they have BCD often take a coal tar B-complex, then wonder why they don't feel any better.

In *Let's Eat Right To Keep Fit,* nutritionist Adelle Davis tells us that many changes in the tongue can alert us to an undersupply of B vitamins. "As the deficiencies of these vitamins become more severe, clumps of taste buds fuse and grow together, pulling apart from other clumps and thus forming grooves and fissures. The first groove usually forms down the center of the tongue. In a severe B-vitamin deficiency, the tongue may be so cut by grooves and fissures that it looks like a relief map of the Grand Canyon and the surrounding territory or a flank steak run through the tenderizing machine." [88]

People who are in a "brain fog" are often deficient in B vitamins. Also, dim vision in the elderly and the red line just under the eyes are symptoms of BCD—vitamin B_2 specifically.

Digestion vs. Indigestion

By now we should all be ready to start eating protein. But then we pause for a moment. What about the heartburn that caused us to stop eating meat in the first place? Or that tendency to feel sluggish after eating, or the uncomfortable sensation of the food just sitting in our stomachs?

Indigestion plagues almost everyone. The top-selling prescribed antacid today is Nexium™, but most people think nothing of popping over-the-counter antacids like Tums™ like candy. "Epigastral reflux" is so common it has become a household term. Where have our digestive systems gone wrong?

Proper digestion enables us to completely break down our food and draw all the nutrients from it. It also helps us stay immune from parasites. In fact, in order to avoid getting candida, we must have plenty of hydrochloric acid (HCl) in our stomachs. The acid portrayed as the "arch-villain" in antacid commercials is **not** HCl, but rather the deviant acids of fermentation. These acids are not the same—at all.

Let's take the digestive process step-by-step. First, you chew your food. This process sends messages to your brain, adrenals, pituitary and other glands to stimulate your stomach to secrete the necessary enzymes to digest the food that's on its way. When the stomach digests, it churns the food along with HCl, juices, pepsin, and enzymes to break it down into chyme. But if there is no HCl the food begins to rot and ferment, much like grapes do when they are used to make wine.

This fermentation process is abnormal to your stomach. It starts churning harder and harder trying to digest the food in it, and sometimes these deviant acids get backed up into the esophagus and cause heartburn. When this goes on for too long, the esophagus can actually be damaged.

What you really need is HCl. To take an antacid at this point ensures that you will have a mass of undigested food left in your stomach, which will then go into your small intestine and put a burden on your gallbladder, liver, and pancreas to try to finish the digestive process . . . and they can't. Your body then begins to get toxic and full of poisons from this undigested matter.

With an undigested food mass decaying and traveling through the 30 feet of the gastrointestinal tract, all kinds of undesirable bacteria and viruses start scavenging this waste. Parasites, which could have been inadvertently swallowed and should have been destroyed by the HCl, are now finding a toxic environment in which to live. *Candida Albicans*, a fungus your body has in place to kill undesirable bacteria, starts to multiply to handle the ever-larger volume of nasty bacteria.

If this sounds disgusting, it is. But the worst part of it is that the body is starting to break down because it is continuously being poisoned. "If you have a concentration of bacteria living in some organ of the body—you have a staph infection or strep in the throat, for instance—they are there because of unhealthy, devitalized tissue and unprocessed metabolic waste. . . . Disease is not the presence of something evil but rather the lack of the presence of something essential." [89]

Eating correctly is important, but digesting what we eat is just as important! Standard Process makes an excellent HCl supplement, Zypan, which also includes pancreatin and pepsin to help the stomach get the job done.

Putting It All Together

This book has been written in an effort to educate you about natural food and soil, whole food supplements vs. synthetic vitamins, and the importance of protein and natural fats in the diet. It is meant to encourage us to go back to the basics of human health. Why? Because it is only in eating the basic diet of our forefathers that our health is truly protected and insured.

Good, whole food is the most important element in our lives. Food is the source of the nutrients required by the human body to perform its many biochemical processes. Without these required nutrients the chemical processes are unable to complete themselves—they peter out. Because nutritional deficiencies are normally not life threatening at first and take time to manifest themselves as serious health problems, many people ignore the early warning signs that their bodies are giving them. Deteriorating joints, depression, and general lethargy are among these warning signs. All too often we dismiss them as being both normal and natural. Worse, we expect them. "Oh, I'm just getting old" is now commonly heard from 30- and 40-year olds.

Many of us just live with health problems and feel that, if we can ignore them, then we're fine. Eventually these become nagging problems we can't ignore. Because of our inattention, existing deficiencies can manifest themselves as patterns of abnormal symptoms and varying degrees of illness. The specific manifestations depend on our state of health to begin with and what sort of foods we put into our bodies every day.

Going back to the basics is a return to foundational nutrition. *Going Back to the Basics* points to the root cause of all symptoms and disease: depleted foods, poor diet, and a sedentary lifestyle. These factors are then further impacted by the negative effect of too much carbohydrate on vitamin and mineral metabolism. The long-term effects of inefficient sugar handling are poor digestion and impaired liver/gallbladder (biliary) function, resulting in a disruption of the endocrine system. This disruption stimulates multiple symptoms and problems, such as the numerous menopausal difficulties women are experiencing today.

Sadly, we must add still other considerations to this picture: toxicity from heavy metals; the toll of decades of substandard foods being produced and consumed, weakening each successive generation; massive amounts of herbicides, pesticides, and fungicides being applied to growing foods; and, to top it all off, literally thousands of untested food additives that are added to processed foods. All of these factors cause the breakdown of our immune systems. Hence, we now have autoimmune diseases we have never heard of before.

Because this has happened over a span of time involving several generations, people have come to accept marginal health as the norm. Think about how much of our modern living and socializing tends to revolve around food—usually junk food— and people eating anything they want. But for most of mankind's time on this planet, people ate to survive and to promote their hardiness. They didn't eat for fun. They ate what nature provided: organ meats and animal fats; fresh, stone-ground whole grains;

raw milk; and dark leafy vegetables (not iceberg lettuce). They ate to keep their bodies strong—which meant their bodies could manufacture the chemical compounds needed by the brain and endocrine system.

As early as 1941 U.S. Surgeon General Dr. Thomas Parran warned in a radio broadcast that " . . . every survey, by whatever method and wherever conducted, shows that malnutrition of many types is widespread and serious among the American people. We eat over-refined foods with most of the natural values processed out of them. Because of this, many well-to-do Americans who can eat what they like are so badly fed as to be physically inferior and mentally dull." [90]

Unfortunately, Dr. Parran's warning was never heeded, and Americans have continually increased their consumption of over-refined foods in every decade since his broadcast. The public has never been given access to **accurate** nutritional information from kindergarten through college. Instead, the processed food industry has been allowed to have its way, and television—with all its commercial sponsors—has served as the main source of nutritional information for the majority of us. Marketing to children has become the processed food industry's forte. Are you aware that "pouring rights" for soda vending machines in schools are now up for the highest bidder?

It is an unhealthy world that we live in. All we can do is start with ourselves. We need to learn the truth and get ourselves and our families healthy first. Then help our friends, gradually working out into our communities and beyond.

How Do We Find The Answers?

In today's health care model, a medical exam usually entails the doctor not touching you and barely taking the time to talk to you, then sending you off for some high-tech testing. Unfortunately, this kind of care has been promoted by HMO business practices that look at the bottom line. Under the influence of drug companies, there is no interest in prevention. The more people get sick and slowly deteriorate, the more money there is to be made. Is it any surprise that so many people find themselves taking several prescriptions a day? In fact, many of our elderly take in excess of a dozen prescriptions daily. We start out with a drug to take care of one symptom; this drug creates side effects that require another drug, and on it goes.

As a result "every day more than 4,000 patients have adverse drug symptoms so serious that they need to be admitted to American hospitals. . . . In addition to the 1.5 million people a year who are admitted to the hospital because of adverse drug reactions, an additional three-quarters of a million people a year develop an adverse drug reaction after they are hospitalized." [91]

The media rarely makes mention of the 100,00 plus people who die each year from adverse drug reactions. These reactions are one of the leading causes of death in America, following heart disease, cancer, and strokes. All of us should have a copy of *Worst Pills, Best Pills: A Consumer Guide to Avoiding Drug-Induced Death or Illness*. This book smoothly guides you through the deadly maze of prescription drug side effects. Is it any wonder so many of us seek alternatives to drugs?

True "health" practitioners are concerned about their patients' lifestyle and diet, which in most cases are the underlying cause of their health problems. Taking this approach is very different from following the traditional medical model, and it requires both action and will power on the part of the patient.

Let's take the example of JoAnn, who has been diagnosed with Chronic Fatigue Syndrome. Every morning on her way to work JoAnn stopped at Starbucks™ for a latte and a sweet roll. By 10 a.m. she would start to feel fatigued, so she would grab a diet soda and a low-calorie candy bar from the vending machine at work. At lunch she would eat a salad because she was trying to be healthy, and she washed it down with another diet soda.

By the time Joann got home she could hardly function. She was too tired to cook for her family, so they regularly grabbed something from a fast food place. Continuing unawares on this path, JoAnn would clearly become a candidate for antidepressants to help her get through the day. But, of course, they wouldn't do a thing for her mounting fatigue. She has a severe blood-sugar handling problem. It is out of control and has been out of control for years. JoAnn is in a vicious cycle and she's starting to pay too high a price.

Let's get JoAnn to an alternative health practitioner who uses the proper tools to analyze her problem—tools that look at function, not pathology. These hands-on tests were part of the training process every doctor received in U.S. medical schools until the 1950s. Although most of these tests could be run and interpreted with accuracy within five minutes, their use was discontinued in favor of machines and new technology many more times expensive and time-consuming to use. This "improved" methodology lacks the personal contact the original tests created between doctor and patient. (We easily forget simplicity and efficiency in our mis-guided quest for the latest improvements in medical technology.)

Lucky for her, JoAnn has found a knowledgeable alternative health practitioner who uses the special tools listed below:

1) **Symptom Survey Questionnaire.** Out of 224 symptoms JoAnn marked 73 of them. The ones checked indicate that she has a severe blood sugar handling problem. Her digestion has been impacted, affecting both pancreatic and gall bladder function.

2) **Nutrition Exam.** When JoAnn's Chapman Reflex point was palpated for pancreatic function, it tested sensitive. When her digestive points were palpated, both showed a need for HCl and pancreatic digestive enzyme support.

3) **Acoustic Cardiograph™ (ACG) Machine.** Based on the original endocardiograph machine invented by Dr. Royal Lee, this machine has a microphone that "listens" to the heartbeat and records the heart function graphically. This is not the same as the EKG, which uses electrical current to measure trauma or damage to the heart. The endocardiograph was used extensively in doctors' offices and clinics throughout the United States from the 1940s to the

1960s. When the ACG was used on JoAnn, the graph showed that she had deficiencies of vitamins B and E. Digestive issues as well as a major adrenal issue also showed up on the graph. The human body will beg, borrow and steal from its reserves to keep the body healthy. If the heart is not functioning optimally, then the body's reserves have been depleted because the food eaten or the supplements that have been taken are not doing the job of maintaining optimum health. (For information about purchasing the ACG call 858-488-2533.)

4) **Reflex Analysis.** There are many reflex systems that have been developed over the last 70 years. Trials matching blood and urine work have proved the accuracy of reflex analysis in determining the cause of many conditions. In JoAnn's case, an advanced non-invasive health analysis was done. (i.e., Nutrition Response Testing (sm) developed by Dr. Freddie Ulan). A thorough exam of this type verified all of her digestive, gall bladder, and adrenal issues as well as her vitamin deficiencies.

With all of this information in place relating to function as root cause, JoAnn is facing a dietary lifestyle change. The alternative health practitioner will recommend whole food supplements to support her digestive, gall bladder, adrenal, and B and E vitamin needs. But, unless she cuts down drastically on her consumption of carbohydrates and sugar, she will not know complete relief or be totally successful in her quest to feel better.

Action Steps

Medical schools train doctors exclusively in allopathic medicine and trauma care. As a result, most doctors overlook prevention and health. Fortunately, the Drs. Eades and others have addressed them both. They have laid out the basics that we all need to know:

1) Eat plenty of protein, ranging from 60-90 grams a day for women and 80-110 grams for men. As much as you can, eat meat free of antibiotics and hormones and organic eggs from free-range chickens. An example of just how important this is comes from Dr. Fred Pescatore's book, *Feed Your Kids Well*. Dr. Pescatore says, "I always tell my patients that organic eggs contain omega-3 and omega-6 fatty acids in the beneficial ratio of one to one. Commercial eggs, on the other hand, contain up to nineteen times more omega-6 than omega-3 fatty acids, making them a very unhealthy product." [92] Also, look for raw milk and raw milk products. Raw milk has gotten a bad rap. Dr. Lee explained, "pasteurized milk is relatively useless as a source of calcium because pasteurization destroys the enzymes that are necessary for the assimilation of the calcium, so insist on raw milk exclusively." [93] No wonder there are so many calcium deficiency-related problems today, from kids whose bones break easily to baby boomers with osteoporosis.

2) Eat plenty of fresh vegetables, especially the green leafy ones, and a limited number of fruits. All of these should be eaten in their whole form, not juiced. Juices are sky-high in carbohydrates and sugar, and many contain high fructose corn syrup (HFCS). (Studies have shown that fructose bypasses your body's regulatory mechanisms and causes insulin levels to rise. USDA researchers autopsied rats that had died after being fed HFCS and found that their livers looked like the livers of alcoholics.) Limit carbohydrate consumption. Eat only whole grains. Try to make sure the produce you purchase is "certified organic." In most cases, this produce contains from 90-250% more nutrients than commercial produce, and a lot fewer pesticides. If organic produce isn't available to you, there are produce cleaners on the market, like Bi-O-Kleen or Organiclean, which help remove pesticides, herbicides, and fungicides from your fruits and vegetables. Also, you

can peel your fruit before you eat it and throw away the outer leaves of leafy vegetables. But really try to get organic produce in your diet. Farmer's markets are springing up all over the country. Mainstream super-markets are beginning to carry more organic foods. It's your life, your health and your world. Stand up for them.

3) Water. Drink a minimum of six to eight glasses a day. (Avoid tap water and drink purified water instead.) Be careful not to drink too <u>much</u> water. This can wash much-needed minerals out of your system.

4) Exercise. Let's face it, you can't be optimally healthy if you just sit or lie around all day long. Get moving! Start to monitor your activity level with a Step-O-Meter. Set a goal for yourself and increase your activity level gradu-ally until you reach your goal. Gardening is great exercise. If you want some structure to increase your level of fitness, Covert Bailey's 1977 book, *Fit or Fat*, is still a reliable guide. He recommends 20 minutes of aerobic exercise at 80% of maximum heart rate three times a week to burn fat and feel better.

5) Consume one to three teaspoons a day of raw olive oil, fresh fish oil, or flax seed oil. Be sure to use butter too.

6) Take adequate amounts of all important vitamins and minerals daily in the form of whole food supplements. Also, be sure to take whatever digestive enzymes you may need. All of the requirements for these should be determined by a health care professional. Remember, whole food supplements are the means for catching up for lost time nutritionally. They are the **only** means.

It is my sincere hope that the information in this book will set you firmly on the path to wellness!

Footnotes

Chapter One

1. Jensen, Bernard, D.C., Ph.D., and Mark Anderson, *Empty Harvest: Understanding the Link Between Our Food, Our Immunity, and Our Planet* (Garden City Park: Avery Publishing Group, 1990), 14.
2. www.gcrio.org [Global Change Research Information Office].
3. www.weru.ksu.edu [Wind Erosion Research Unit].
4. von Liebig, Baron Justus, *The Natural Laws of Husbandry,* ed. John Blyth, M.D. (London: Walton & Maberly, 1863).
5. Jensen and Anderson, *op. cit.*, 75.
6. Howard, Albert, *An Agricultural Testament* (Emmaus, PA: Rodale Press, 1973).
7. Jensen and Anderson, *Empty Harvest*, 32.
8. *Ibid.*, 57.
9. *New Yorker* magazine, 10 April 2000, 58.
10. Jensen and Anderson, *op. cit.*, 46-47.
11. *Ibid.*, 8.
12. *Ibid.*, 55.
13. *Ibid.*, 7.
14. *Ibid.*, 27.
15. *Ibid.*
16. *Ibid.*, 97.
17. *Ibid.*, 37.
18. Wiley, Harvey W., M.D., *The History of a Crime Against the Food Law: The Amazing Story of the National Food and Drugs Law Intended to Protect the Health of the People Perverted to Protect Adulteration of Foods and Drugs* (Washington, D.C.: Harvey W. Wiley, 1929), 391.
19. *Ibid.*, 401-402.
20. *Washington Post*, 26 October 1949.
21. *Celebrating 75 Years: The History of Standard Process Inc. 1929-2004* (Palmyra, WI: Standard Process Inc., 2004).
22. Jensen and Anderson, *op. cit.*, 38.
23. *Ibid.*
24. *Ibid.*, 39.
25. *Ibid.*, 36.

26.   Senate Committee on the Judiciary, "Invasions of Privacy
        (Government Agencies)," Hearings on SR 39 Part 2, 89th Congress,
        1st session (19 April–7 June 1965), 739.
27.   Jensen and Anderson, *op. cit.*, 126-127.
28.   DeCava, Judith A., *The Real Truth about Vitamins and Antioxidants*
        (West Yarmouth, MA: A Printery, 1997), 139.
29.   www.MSNBC.com [MSNBC News Service], 5 December 2006.
30.   Enig, Mary G., PhD., *Know Your Fats: The Complete Primer for
        Understanding the Nutrition of Fats, Oils, and Cholesterol* (Silver
        Springs, MD: Bethesda Press, 2000), 86.
31.   Lee, Royal, D.D.S., *Lectures of Dr. Royal Lee Vol. 1*, ed. Mark R.
        Anderson (Fort Collins, CO: Selene River Press, 1998), 143.
32.   www.fluoridealert.org.
33.   *The Merck Manual of Medical Information (Home Edition),* ed.
        Robert Berkow, M.D. (Whitehouse Station, NJ: Merck Research
        Laboratories, 1997), 709.

Chapter Two

34.   DeCava, Judith A., *The Real Truth about Vitamins and Antioxidants*
        (West Yarmouth, MA: A Printery, 1997), 37.
35.   *Ibid.*, p. 38.
36.   *Ibid.*
37.   Cheraskin, Emanuel, and W.M. Ringsdorf, *New Hope for Incurable
        Diseases* (Jericho, NY: Exposition Press, Inc., 1973), 83-85.
38.   DeCava, *op. cit.*, 37.
39.   Horrobin, D. F., *The Philosophical Basis of Peer Review and the
        Suppression of Innovation* (JAMA, March 1990), 1439-1440.
40.   Krause, Marie V., and Kathleen Mahan, *Food, Nutrition and Diet
        Therapy* (Philadelphia: W.B. Saunders Company, 1979), 148-149.
41.   *Taber's Cyclopedic Medical Dictionary*, ed. Clayton Thomas, M.D.
        (Philadelphia: F.A. Davis Company, 1985).
42.   *Ibid.*, 15.
43.   *Ibid.*, 57.
44.   *Ibid.*, 59.
45.   Lee, Royal, D.D.S., *Vitamin News Vol. 8*, 135.
46.   DeCava, *op. cit.*, 54.
47.   *Ibid.*, 117.
48.   *Ibid.*, 119.
49.   *Ibid.*, 163.
50.   *Ibid.*, 190.
51.   Jensen, Bernard, D.C., Ph.D., and Mark Anderson, *Empty Harvest:*

Understanding the Link Between Our Food, Our Immunity, and Our Planet (Garden City Park: Avery Publishing Group, 1990), 123.

52. DeCava, *op. cit.*, 64.
53. Toufexis, Anastasia, *Time Magazine*, 6 April 1992, 54-59.
54. DeCava, *op. cit.*, 70.
55. Challem, Jack, "Are You Overdoing Antioxidants?" *Natural Health Vol. 25:3*, May/June 1995, 56-57.
56. Jensen and Anderson, *op. cit.*, 25.
57. *Ibid.*, 47.
58. *Ibid.*
59. Murray, Richard P., D.C., 1995, Natural vs. synthetic, life vs. death, truth vs. the lie, published by author, 4.
60. *Ibid.*
61. *Ibid.*, 5.
62. West, Bruce, M.D., "Do Your Supplements Cause Indigestion?" *Health Alert Vol. 14:3*, March 1997.
63. Rodale, J.I. and Staff, *The Complete Book of Food and Nutrition* (Emmaus, PA: Rodale Books, 1961) quoted in *Empty Harvest* (Garden City Park: Avery Publishing Group, 1990), 127-128.

Chapter Three

64. Levenstein, Harvey, *Revolution at the Table: The Transformation of the American Diet* (New York: Oxford University Press, 1988), 33.
65. *Ibid.*, 34.
66. Eades, Michael R., M.D., and Mary Dan Eades, M.D., *Protein Power* (New York: Bantam Books, 1996), 36.
67. Taubes, Gary, "The Soft Science of Dietary Fat," *Science Vol. 291:5513*, 30 March 2001, 2536-2545.
68. *Ibid.*
69. *Ibid.*
70. *Ibid.*
71. Taubes, Gary, "What If It's All Been A Big Fat Lie?" *New York Times,* 7 July 2002.
72. Taubes, Gary, "The Soft Science of Dietary Fat," *op. cit.*
73. Levenstein, Harvey, *Paradox of Plenty: A Social History of Eating in Modern America* (New York: Oxford University Press, 1993), 106.
74. Lee, Royal, D.D.S., *Lectures of Dr. Royal Lee Vol. 1*, ed. Mark R. Anderson (Fort Collins, CO: Selene River Press, 1998), 65.
75. Sears, Barry, Ph.D., with Bill Lawren, *Enter the Zone: A Dietary Road Map* (New York: Regan Books/HarperCollins, 1995), 8.
76. Eades and Eades, *op. cit.*, 61.

77. *Ibid.*, 41.
78. *Ibid.*
79. *Ibid.*, 92-93.
80. *Ibid.*, 99.
81. *Ibid.*, 58.
82. House Committee on Government Reform, Subcommittee on Human Rights and Wellness, Testimony of Eric H. Bost (Under Secretary Food, Nutrition and Consumer Services), 15 September 2004.
83. Eades and Eades, *op. cit.*, 62.
84. Abramson, John, M.D., *Overdosed America: The Broken Promise of American Medicine* (New York: Harper Perennial, 2005), 132.
85. Sears, Barry, Ph.D., *op. cit.*, 32.

Chapter Four

86. Pottenger, Francis M. Jr., M.D., *Pottenger's Cats: A Study in Nutrition* (San Diego, CA: Price-Pottenger Nutrition Foundation, 1983), 93.
87. *Ibid.*
88. Davis, Adelle, *Let's Eat Right to Keep Fit* (New York: Harcourt Brace Jovannovich, Inc., 1970), 66.
89. Jensen, Bernard, D.C., Ph.D., and Mark Anderson, *Empty Harvest: Understanding the Link Between Our Food, Our Immunity, and Our Planet* (Garden City Park: Avery Publishing Group, 1990), 113.
90. *Ibid.*
91. Wolfe, Sidney M., M.D., et al., *Worst Pills, Best Pills: A Consumer's Guide to Avoiding Drug-Induced Death or Illness* (New York: Pocket Books/Simon and Schuster, Inc., 2005), 10.
92. Pescatore, Fred, M.D., *Feed Your Kids Well: How to Help Your Child Lose Weight and Get Healthy* (New York: John Wiley & Sons, Inc., 1998), 84.
93. Lee, Royal, D.D.S., *Lectures of Dr. Royal Lee Vol. 1*, ed. Mark R. Anderson (Fort Collins, CO: Selene River Press, 1998), 17.

"Your body is deficient in vitamins, minerals, enzymes, and cofactors. That is a fact. There is no way that you can get all the nutrients you need by eating food. You would have to eat ten to twenty times the amount of food as you are now, and it would all have to be organic. There is simply no way you are getting the nutrients you need. . . . I suggest buying a whole food concentrate nutritional supplement."

Kevin Trudeau
Natural Cures "They" Don't Want You To Know About

Resources

All of the materials referenced in this book are highly recommended readings.

The International Foundation for Nutrition and Health: (858) 488-8932 and www.ifnh.org. The foundation has been entrusted with the stewardship of the original materials by Dr. Royal Lee, Dr. Harrower, Dr. Page, and Dr. Hawkins, as well as other classic works in nutrition.

Fluoridation: The Great Dilemma by G.L. Waldbott, A.W. Burgstahler, and H.L. McKinney, Coronado Press Inc. © 1978.

Natural Cures "They" Don't Want You To Know About by Kevin Trudeau, Alliance Publishing Group, Inc., © 2004.

Book Editing: Mo Rafael, Bright Earth Books, (760) 402-1128, brightearth@safe-mail.net

Index

A

B

C

Howard, Sir Albert, 8
hormone, 65
human annihilation, 15
hydrochloric acid (HCl), 74
hydrogenated, 16, 24
hypoglycemia, 64, 72

I

immune disorders, 26
indigestion, 73, 74
infant mortality rate (U.S.),
    24, 72
insomnia, 73
insulin, 64, 65, 66, 67, 68, 69,
    70, 81
irregular heart beat, 73
iron, 3, 14
irradiated ergosterol, 38

J

JAMA, 28
Jarvis, DC, 42
junk food, 76

K

Kellogg's, 56
Keys, Ancel, 60, 61

L

LDL cholesterol, 68
lecithin, 24
Lee, Dr. Royal, 19, 20, 22, 23,
    24, 27, 38, 39, 49, 50, 51,
    52, 53, 63, 79
Let's Eat Right to Keep Fit, 73

Levenstein, Harvey, 55, 61
Liebig, Baron Justus von, 8
life expectancy, 1, 2
liver, 76
lobbying, 28
low birth weight, 26
low-fat diets, 3, 55, 56, 57, 59,
    60

M

manganese, 71
Manura, J.J., 24
mainstream nutritional
    science, 57
McCoy, Clive, 62
McGovern, Senator George,
    59, 60
medical schools, 31, 32
Mellon Institute, 27
mental confusion, 73
Merck, 32
metabolic procescesses, 45
micrograms, 31, 40
milligrams, 31, 39, 40
modern agriculture, 10
molecular complexity, 39
Morgan, Agnes Faye, 19
Mother Jones Magazine, 12
Murray, Richard P., 51

N

natural vitamins, 30, 34
Nazi Germany, 53
Nelson, Elmer M., 19
New York City Board of
    Health, 26
niacin, 30, 39

NOTES

NOTES

NOTES

NOTES

Ode To A Shelf-Life

Ah, but to last longer on the shelf
It certainly has made an industry of wealth
To enrich, store and transport has been the goal
My body doesn't know the difference, I am told
If I could but last as long as thee,
Oh odorless oils, canned foods, cereal and candy

—Anonymous